PRAISE FOR LONGEVITY MADE SIMPLE

"Want to add years to your life and life to your years? To live longer and better? Here's how! Elegantly and clearly written by renowned experts who understand healthy living so well, they can make it simple. Highly recommended!"

—Dean Ornish, M.D.
#1 New York Times bestselling author
Clinical Professor of Medicine, UCSF

"As a physician deeply committed to root-cause medicine and transforming our broken healthcare system into one that promotes true health, I am thrilled to see a book like *Longevity Made Simple* enter the world. Dr. Shad and Dr. Carmona, two leading voices in preventive medicine and public health, have written an inspiring and accessible roadmap for how we can live healthier, longer lives.

Their DRESS Code—Diet, Relationships, Exercise, Stress, and Sleep—is more than just an acronym. It is a science-based, lifestyle-first framework for rewiring how we think about health, aging, and disease. Drawing from real patient stories, cutting-edge research on epigenetics and lifestyle medicine, and decades of clinical and public health leadership, this book powerfully bridges the gap between what we know and what we do.

In a time when most healthcare is focused on reactive disease management, this book empowers individuals to take control of their biology, upgrade their habits, and extend not just their lifespan but their healthspan. Longevity Made Simple is essential reading for anyone who wants to prevent disease, reverse chronic conditions, and unlock their fullest potential. This book is a must-read for anyone who wants to live not just longer, but better."

—Dr. Mark Hyman,
Co-founder & Chief Medical Officer
and author of the #1 New York Times bestseller, *Young Forever*

"*Longevity Made Simple* is a compelling and practical guide to living better for longer. Dr. Shad Marvasti and Dr. Richard Carmona have masterfully distilled the complex science of epigenetics to explain the foundational lifestyle principles we uncovered in the world's longest-lived communities into actionable strategies for everyday life. The DRESS Code offers a clear, structured path to better health, empowering readers from all walks of life to take small, sustainable steps toward a longer, more meaningful life. It's an inspiring companion for anyone who wants to live a longer, happier life with more vitality, joy, and purpose. This book is both a science-based roadmap and an invitation—to take control of your health and thrive."

—Dan Buettner,
Founder of the Blue Zones and
#1 New York Times bestselling author

"*Longevity Made Simple* is both medically sound and deeply human. Dr. Shad and Dr. Carmona bring years of clinical expertise and public health leadership to a message that is as inspiring as it is actionable. Through the DRESS Code—Diet, Relationships, Exercise, Stress, and Sleep—readers will receive a proven, science-based path to prevent disease and extend not just their lifespan, but their healthspan. This book is a much-needed guide for anyone who wants to take charge of their health and live with greater clarity, vitality, and purpose."

—Dr. Sanjay Gupta,
CNN Chief Medical Correspondent, Neurosurgeon,
and #1 Bestselling Author of Keep Sharp

Who doesn't want to live healthier for longer?! Dr. Shad and Dr. Carmona have done a masterful job of making the message of lifestyle medicine—evidence-based, therapeutic lifestyle change—simple and digestible by giving us a DRESS Code that equips and empowers each of us to add years to life and life to years. The book emphasizes that our genes are not our destiny: Evidence shows that the choices we make each and every day about what we eat, how we move, how we think, and other DRESS Code "lifestyle medicine pillars" have the power to protect our health and fight disease, slowing down and even reversing the aging process. The vision of a nation and world filled with Blue Zones will manifest when we—physicians, healthcare professionals, and patients alike—prescribe, embrace, and adopt the DRESS Code outlined herein. And what a beautiful world it will be!

—Susan Benigas,
Chief Executive Officer at The American College
of Lifestyle Medicine

"*Longevity Made Simple* is a timely and transformative contribution to the future of health and well-being. Dr. Shad and Dr. Carmona have shared the latest science and real-world clinical experience in the form of an accessible framework—the DRESS Code—that is both practical and profoundly empowering. This book aligns perfectly with the mission we champion at the Lake Nona Impact Forum: to shift from reactive care to proactive, personalized, and preventative health strategies that help communities and individuals thrive. It's a must-read for anyone working to create healthier, more resilient lives and systems."

—Gloria Caulfield,
Founder and Executive Director,
Lake Nona Impact Forum, President, Lake Nona Institute

"Longevity has suddenly become an overly complex, confusing and expensive pursuit. In all my decades in the wellness space, this book provides the most dazzlingly simple—but most science-backed—roadmap to living healthier and longer. By focusing on the DRESS code—making very doable changes in your diet, relationships, exercise, sleep and stress—you can achieve a powerful epigenetic 'reset,' literally turning on or off thousands of your genes in just a few weeks. You don't need to be a billionaire to biohack your healthspan, you just need this book."

—Susie Ellis,
Chairman and CEO of the Global Wellness Institute

Longevity

Made Simple:

Live Healthier for Longer
with the DRESS Code

Shad Marvasti, MD, MPH

with Richard H. Carmona, MD, MPH

Foreword by Andrew Weil, MD

A POST HILL PRESS BOOK
ISBN: 979-8-89565-588-7
ISBN (eBook): 979-8-89565-589-4

Cover design by Julia Kuris
Copyediting by Claudia Volkman
Interior & eBook design by Amit Dey
Author photo by Byron Medina

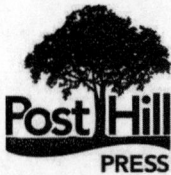

Post Hill Press
New York • Nashville
posthillpress.com

Published in the United States of America
1 2 3 4 5 6 7 8 9 10

To the loving memory of my mother who taught me the incredible power of faith, and to my dear father who has always believed in me and inspired me to aim high in my service to humanity in all that I do. To my dear wife, Shahrzad, who is my best friend and the love of my life, who selflessly gives our family all the time, guidance, wisdom, and support that we need to thrive. And to our boys, Darian, Kamdin, and Aran who have taught me how to be a father and continue to enrich my life with their love and enthusiasm in discovering new adventures every day.

CONTENTS

PREFACE

For most of my life, I have been a first responder, from routine trauma and emergency care to combat casualty care and catastrophic events such as hurricanes, earthquakes, tsunamis, terrorist events, and, now, a pandemic.

As an ocean lifeguard, Army Special Forces combat medic "operator," paramedic, registered nurse, police officer, trauma surgeon, and emergency medical system director, the quest to save lives was exhilarating, but never enough. Over the years, I realized that most of the conditions I treated were preventable. Whether it is people becoming sedentary and adding to a growing obesity epidemic fueled by poor eating habits, an explosion of preventable chronic diseases, or escalating trauma from gun violence or other causes, what has become glaringly evident to me is that the trajectory our nation is on is unsustainable. We are drowning in preventable disease and economic burden. US healthcare spending continues to grow alarmingly, and now costs us more than $4 trillion annually, or approximately 18 percent of our GDP. This is by far the highest expenditure of all developed countries, and yet our health outcomes are not the best. We also know that, besides our healthcare system being unsustainable, we spend approximately seventy-five to eighty cents of every US "healthcare" dollar on treating preventable diseases related to poor lifestyle choices. In effect, we have a struggling "sick care" system, not a "healthcare" system.

Two decades ago, I began migrating toward public health and prevention. As a professor, I went back to grad school to get a master's degree in public health policy and administration. I eventually became the CEO of the local county hospital and healthcare system, which included the Public Health Department.

As I found a new home in public health and left the daily media-driven drama of saving lives behind me, I realized how odd it was that the public health endeavors that saved populations rarely got the media attention they deserved.

After several years at the helm of our public healthcare system along the US-Mexico border, I had the privilege and opportunity to return to uniformed active service as the United States Surgeon General.

After completing my statutory term as the Surgeon General, I once again returned to civilian life and fully committed myself to national and global public health endeavors in academics and the private business sector. Reflecting on my life trajectory, I now realize that some of my best "training" and experience was growing up poor and living in the "hood" of Harlem, New York City, as the oldest son of poor emigrant parents whose second language was English.

In retrospect, my life and my family's was the antithesis of the DRESS Code that we offer in this book. Being poor, at times homeless, and not having ready access to health and dental care or a secure wholesome food chain defined our lives. Unfortunately, this scenario continues globally, and, remarkably, in the richest country in the world, our own United States.

Albert Einstein once stated that we should not expect different outcomes if we keep doing the same thing. Therefore, we must disrupt the status quo and embrace the DRESS Code. Failure is not an option, for the preservation of humanity is at stake.

Ironically, most of what I know about the DRESS Code is based on the traditions and culture passed down to me by my ancestors, especially my grandmother, a.k.a. Abuelita. My decades in higher education after being a high school dropout provided me with the scientific knowledge I needed to validate the practices that Abuelita and our ancestors had taught me.

I remember being told as a child to go out and play, be nice to others, make friends, eat your "greens," and get a good night's sleep. Each of the aforementioned we know today as epigenetic inputs, which are actions that code and recode your genes to optimize gene expression or function. How intuitively correct our ancestors were! Now, we can explain their guidance on a genetic and molecular level through cultural traditions.

Abuelita knew and practiced the DRESS Code at a macro level. In effect, the DRESS Code comprises dependent variables, which, if practiced, will help you feel younger, and live a longer, happier, healthier, cheaper life! In those "Blue Zones," where it is common to become a healthy, mobile centenarian, we find that these and other epigenetic inputs are common, essential, and the true Fountain of Youth. Ironically, it is the departure from our ancestral DRESS Code that has caused the growing preventable disease and economic burden. Now we must go back to our future!

As we relearn the elements of the DRESS Code, the evolving multidisciplinary science also allows us to create a world driven by precision health and wellness. Knowing your genome and applying evolving science, such as nutrigenomics, pharmacogenomics, and psychogenomics, will allow you in the future to choose precise epigenetic inputs that will optimize your gene expression and your human performance. The simplicity of the acronym of the DRESS Code belies its importance in our lives.

As we forensically dissect the components of the DRESS Code: diet, relationships, exercise, stress, and sleep, I continue to marvel at how our ancestors, without advanced scientific tools, arrived at these life-dependent variables.

—Richard H. Carmona, MD, MPH, FACS

FOREWORD
by Andrew Weil, MD

I met Dr. Shad when he was a medical student: I was impressed with his interest in changing the way medicine is practiced, which he has continued to implement when treating patients and educating colleagues and the general public. Dr. Carmona is a long-time friend and a popular lecturer to classes of physician Fellows at the Andrew Weil University of Arizona Center for Integrative Medicine. Drs. Shad's and Carmona's attitudes toward health and wellness are completely aligned with my own views and with Integrative Medicine philosophy.

Despite all that has been written by me and others on natural health, natural medicine, and the importance of eating better to improve one's health and longevity, there are still so many preventable deaths in the United States, which now lags behind most other developed countries in health outcomes. In 2020, driven by the COVID-19 pandemic, life expectancy in the U.S. dropped to 77.3 years, compared to an average of 82 in these comparable countries. Premature death rates and disease burden in the U.S. are higher than in comparable countries, and the U.S. ranks last among them in measures of healthcare access and quality.[1] How has this happened?

Drs. Shad and Carmona have witnessed this decline firsthand, and they have had success using the DRESS Code to help their patients improve their health and increase their potential longevity. The DRESS Code is a simple acronym for Diet, Relationships,

Exercise, Stress, and Sleep—which are the key components to living a healthier life. The authors of this book are committed to educating not only their own patients but anyone who is interested in living not only longer but *better.*

Like them, I believe that health is an individual responsibility. As I wrote in *Why Our Health Matters*, it's up to you to learn how to maintain your own health and protect your body's healing potential as you go through life. In fact, the basic tenet of Integrative Medicine is that the human body can heal itself. Many of my other books have focused on the importance of eating well for optimum health; Drs. Shad and Carmona provide the specific guidance you need to make positive life changes, prevent illness, and maintain wellness not only by attending to diet but also to other critical factors. Written in easy-to-understand language for readers who are *not* doctors or scientists, this book explains what *you* can do to protect your health and overall well-being, including advice about improving relationships, exercise habits (even if you don't have any yet!), stress management, and sleep.

I recommend this book to readers of all ages.

— Andrew Weil, MD

INTRODUCTION

I was exhausted. I had been up for nearly thirty-five hours. I briefly paused and went to the bathroom to gather myself before presenting at a noon conference. I looked at my sunken, tired eyes in the mirror. How was I even standing? Why is the process of becoming a full-fledged doctor so painful and so unhealthy? My thoughts then wandered again to what had happened the night before. As I looked down at my hands in the sink, I couldn't believe what I had done over the last day.

It started out routinely with breakfast and driving in to work. Then, it started. One patient after another, one with a heart attack, another with a stroke, then two babies to deliver back-to-back and a code blue to oversee. And it kept going on from there, with more patient admissions to the hospital than I care to remember. This was a day in the life of my experience as a medical resident. I learned a great deal from an amazing group of expert physicians. I saw patient after patient with heart attacks, strokes, heart failure, complications from cancer, diabetic comas, and all sorts of emergencies. The pace of work was draining and overwhelming, without enough time to process what was happening.

When I did have some downtime in between shifts or on a day off, I began to reflect on the types of conditions we treated. I realized that we kept seeing the same people coming in and out of the hospital, only to come back again a few weeks or a couple months later. And these people were not always old; many were in their fifties or sixties, and some were much younger than that. What they all had in common was a chronic disease—one that gradually debilitated them, kept them sick, and kept them coming back, again and again. How was this healthcare? We were definitely saving people in acute crisis, which was rewarding, but we weren't making people better by solving the root causes of their diseases.

I started to realize that our job as physicians was to "stabilize" people so they could walk, eat, and go to the bathroom before releasing them back into the wild, only to see them return again soon after. Why would this happen? Was this going to be the main focus of my life as a physician—temporarily putting people together, only to have them remain half-sick until their next hospitalization? Was this simply inevitable for everyone? Do we have to develop diabetes, high cholesterol, or blood pressure, or become overweight and develop some chronic disease that keeps us from living our best life?

Well, the statistics show a grim picture, both then and now. According to the CDC, six out of ten Americans suffer from a chronic disease. And when we look at what chronic conditions people are suffering from, it is the same major disease categories both in the United States and around the world: cardiovascular disease, diabetes, cancer, obesity, non-infectious airway diseases like asthma or COPD, and various forms of dementia. In the United States, these conditions have consistently accounted for nearly 80 percent of all healthcare expenditures and seven out of ten deaths. Globally, chronic disease has outpaced acute infectious disease and is now responsible for over 60 percent of all global deaths.

Even with the acute infectious COVID-19 pandemic, the people who had one of these chronic diseases or risk factors for them, like high blood pressure, were at higher risk for more severe disease, hospitalization, and death from an acute COVID infection. Chances are, most of you reading this book are directly impacted by or have a risk factor for one of these conditions or have a family member or friend with one of these chronic diseases.

Going back to my time as a resident at Stanford, the question that kept coming back to my mind was: Is this all inevitable? Was there something we could do to prevent this from happening? Could we not find and address the root causes of these conditions? I thought to myself that if this was all that we could do, then what, other than comforting and connecting with people, are we really doing here? Just keeping people alive with limited ability to live a full, functional life seemed like a bleak prospect. I needed to know that there was more. I needed to understand why this was happening and what could be done to prevent it.

I remember one patient, Miguel. Miguel was forty-six years old when I first met him. He had been diagnosed with type 2 diabetes five years before we met, and when I saw him, he had suffered his second acute diabetic coma in the last four years. He was married with three children and had a deep love for his family, who also immensely loved him. His family history was not only positive for diabetes, but also for heart disease and premature heart attack; his father had died at age fifty-three. Diabetes is a known risk factor for heart disease. After working with the team to save Miguel from his second life-threatening diabetes coma and stabilizing his condition, we spent some time talking. When he was discharged from the hospital, he became my patient. As a family medicine physician, I had the privilege of also taking care of his wife and children. I learned about their lives—their faith, their cultural practices, their diet, and their lifestyles. I also learned that Miguel believed he was destined to have diabetes and was afraid that he too would die prematurely of a heart attack, like his father. I didn't want to accept this. No one should have to accept this.

Diabetes is not a death sentence. Despite this, it has been for far too long and for far too many people. Diabetes is the leading cause of lower limb amputation, non-congenital blindness, and kidney failure in the United States. All these tragic consequences happen as a result of excessively high blood sugar levels.

Around 95 percent of diabetes cases are type 2 diabetes, which is caused by insulin resistance. Insulin resistance is not a genetically inherited condition. Insulin resistance is caused by a combination of lifestyle factors, such as a poor diet and sedentary or inactive lifestyle. It can be prevented, and, in many instances, even be reversed. And that's what I told Miguel and his family. Not surprisingly, I was the first doctor to tell them this. That's because, as physicians, we are trained to treat disease as part of a reactive disease management system. We are highly skilled in dealing with an acute crisis, yet we learn far too little about prevention or how to keep patients healthy. Instead, we are focused on what to do with them when they are sick. Our treatment is mostly focused on medication and surgery, with little, if any, practical advice about diet, exercise, or any meaningful lifestyle changes to keep us healthy. In this regard, I've always been inclined to the path less traveled by most in healthcare, as I was exposed to a different perspective from an early age. My own life experiences prompted me to take a different approach to caring for Miguel and other patients like him.

Growing up as an immigrant in the United States, I saw how my parents balanced the traditions of our heritage with the prevailing narrative of our new home, especially when it came to healthcare. We believed in the importance of medicine when battling illness, but my mother had also studied nutrition and always believed in the use of food as medicine; my father, an accountant by profession, shared my mother's views on food and cultural practices to stay healthy as a first line remedy for many ailments.

Drawing on eating practices from my culture, which originated from the ancient Persian medicine of the Old Silk Road, I always knew what foods were "warm-natured" (honey or ginger) and what foods were "cold-natured" (watermelon and cucumber), and why it was important to balance these to maintain health. Sometimes, when I would get sick, my parents would suggest that I was *saardi* or overly cold from eating too many cold-natured foods. They would give me a few warm-natured foods, and I would miraculously feel better. Beyond food, I also learned about other practices to maintain health, including meditation and prayer to stay focused on what matters in life, the importance of getting quality sleep, and why movement is a key part of well-being. These childhood experiences and lifestyle practices passed on to me by my parents have stayed with me throughout my life.

When I was twelve years old, I experienced the power of manual medicine and herbal remedies that prevented me from getting what we realized later was an unnecessary surgery suggested by conventional doctors. While this was a remarkable experience for me and pointed me toward the potential impact of complementary and alternative medicine, I knew there was value to conventional care as well.

Several years later, when I was nineteen years old, I witnessed the power of surgery to save my mother's life through a kidney transplant—a miracle of modern science. I didn't understand why these different, yet complementary, approaches couldn't be used in medicine as part of a balanced approach to keeping us all healthy. Why couldn't medicine do both? Why do we have to limit ourselves to medication or surgery, when there are so many other options, including food as medicine and lifestyle changes, to prevent and treat our illnesses?

To answer these questions, I decided to engage in research on these lifestyle-based approaches, and quickly realized I was not alone in this interest. It was at this point that I discovered Dr. Andrew Weil's books on integrative medicine. I saw in integrative medicine an inspiring approach to health and medicine that embraced the best of both worlds to address the diseases of our time with a holistic focus on prevention and wellness.

In the summer of 1997, I decided to apply these intellectual insights to initiate a research internship in the Complementary and Alternative Medicine Program at Stanford, known as CAMPS. Having recently engaged in humanities research on the history of medicine, I was surprised that a prestigious university such as Stanford was researching unconventional approaches like tai chi for blood pressure management and garlic for high cholesterol. I quickly learned how much evidence was building for these age-old remedies or practices, and how much more research was needed to ultimately integrate these cost-effective and safe therapies into conventional medicine.

Between Dr. Weil's books and my research, I recognized that our system was still focusing on an acute care model, a narrow and outdated approach using episodic care to treat symptoms of disease without an emphasis on prevention or health. I also realized that health disparities and existing policies are contributing to the development of the chronic diseases of our time.

My insight was confirmed when I worked as a community organizer with the health department in Guadalupe, Arizona, a land-locked town in the middle of urban Phoenix, surrounded by freeways and other cities. The town had a rich cultural history from both the Yaqui Indians and Mexican American traditions, yet it is disproportionately challenged by poverty and chronic diseases like diabetes.

During my time volunteering and working in the community, I learned about the social-level determinants of health and witnessed firsthand how the way we live impacts our ability to make healthy choices to prevent disease. I also witnessed how these factors negatively contribute to health disparities and lack of equal access to high-quality healthcare. Based on these experiences, I decided that, for me, it was just as important to learn about the role of public health in preventing disease as it was to understand the role of individual patient decisions in this process. I realized that public policies could set us up for failure or for success.

For patients like Manual and his family, living on a limited income meant they had to decide between paying basic bills and paying for food. Because of federal subsidies in the Farm Bill, millions of families like Manual's family are left with difficult choices, as the cheapest food options are the unhealthiest. In fact, people who have Supplemental Nutrition Assistance Program (SNAP) benefits popularly known as "food stamps" are more likely to be obese and diabetic. That's because the number one product that is currently purchased in this program is soda. This was also the case for Manual and his family, which is why we had to identify resources to help them make better choices. It was disheartening for me to see how challenging it was for people to make the healthy choice.

This, combined with the sheer volume of people sick with preventable chronic diseases, including diabetes or heart disease, weighed heavily on me as a physician-in-training. I reflected on how lifestyle practices were so critical for health, yet so underutilized by medical doctors to prevent, treat, and even reverse these chronic conditions. I was filled with a desire to learn more about the science behind food and lifestyle to change the practice of medicine.

And that's the perspective I had when I was caring for Miguel and his family. I started to share some of my experiences and thoughts about disease prevention. I talked about how having a family history of diabetes or heart disease did not mean that everyone in that family would be fated to have it. Things could be done. The heart attack that Manual and his family feared was not inevitable. Gradually, we began to identify components of Miguel's diet and lifestyle that were contributing to his uncontrolled diabetes. Like many of us, his diet included many processed foods that are sadly both cheap and widely available. When you are a family of five, the cost of food can be a big barrier to eating healthy. But thankfully, there are opportunities even for families like Miguel's, who were also using food stamps to get by.

I was able to connect them with a local program that, years later, evolved into the Double Up Food Bucks program. This program essentially doubled the buying power of food stamps in local farmers' markets. In addition to resources like these, we also discussed how exactly to use these foods and create specific diets in the form of a food prescription to treat Miguel's diabetes. We also discussed how these same whole, real foods could also decrease his risk for a heart attack by stabilizing his blood pressure and lowering his bad cholesterol.

After working with him for a year, Manual's sugars started to come down and stay down. When I first met him, he was on insulin and three different medications for diabetes. After six months, he was down to half the insulin and two medications. By a year, he had lost forty-five pounds, and his blood sugar was now in the prediabetes range. His blood pressure was normal (not requiring the two blood pressure medications he was on previously) and so was his cholesterol, without the need for a statin medication. Since I always asked for his wife to be present at the visits (as I would see her and their kids as patients all together), she also made lifestyle changes that resulted in weight loss and a reversal of her prediabetes status. This was exciting for Miguel, his wife, and their family. No more visits to the hospital for diabetic comas or fear of a heart attack looming in the future.

Miguel's case is not atypical. In fact, since residency, I have had the privilege of caring for many people with similar challenges. And in every situation, I've witnessed the power of lifestyle to prevent and even reverse chronic conditions like type 2 diabetes and heart disease.

In learning more about the science behind these clinical success stories with my patients, I have come to understand that the genes we inherit at birth are not our destiny.

Our genes are not our destiny.

The idea that the chronic conditions that now account for seven out of every ten deaths and more than 77 percent of all health expenditures in the United States are predetermined by our genes is simply false. Genes are part of the story and play a role. But how much of a role do they play? It turns out that genes only contribute between 20 to 30 percent of our total risk for the development of the chronic diseases of our time. The lion's share of our risk for these conditions is not our genes—it's our lifestyle and the society we live in. We now know that our zip code is far more impactful than our genetic code. Where we live, how we live, how we play, whom we connect with—these social, behavioral, and lifestyle factors are the key determinants of health.

To go further, the science of epigenetics confirms how these factors play out at the molecular level to change our fate by changing the expression of our genes. Epigenetics literally translates to the study of what is above and beyond our genes. While there are conditions that are strongly determined by genes, the vast majority of the chronic conditions we now face are not. These conditions arise from many genes and how they interact with the world through what we do and what we are exposed to. Epigenetics is the study of how these interactions change the expression of our genes for better or for worse. For example, the field of nutrigenomics (epigenetics of nutrition) is now demonstrating the power of food as medicine.

Epigenetics is the study of how these interactions change the expression of our genes for better or for worse. For example, the field of nutrigenomics (epigenetics of nutrition) is now demonstrating the power of food as medicine.

While this is an ancient concept practiced for thousands of years across the globe, we are now recognizing the molecular impact of food as a messenger signal to the genes in our cells. Our diet is like information that can literally turn on or off thousands of genes in a matter of weeks. That's right—not years or even months, but *weeks*.

And certain real foods, acting as epigenetic inputs, can optimize our health by turning on the protective genes and turning off the genes that increase our risk for disease.

While diet is a critical factor, it is not the only epigenetic input that drives health or disease; there are several others that we will focus on in this book. The same can be said for exercise, stress, relationships, and sleep.

While there are many opinions on how to live longer, which can make it seem complicated, it is clear that optimizing our lifestyle is the most important thing we can do. In this book, we will explore how the key areas of lifestyle help us live a longer, healthier life. The acronym DRESS, as envisioned by Dr. Carmona, encapsulates these key elements of lifestyle:

D=Diet

R=Relationships

E=Exercise

S=Sleep

S=Stress

Imagine you are attending a formal event with a strict dress code. This is a VIP-only experience, where all you need to do is show up wearing the right clothes that fit the code. If you do not comply, you will not be allowed in and will miss out on all the joys and benefits of the event (this could be a special party, dining at a restaurant or going to the opera, or any other special gathering). In the same way, getting access to the VIP experience in life also requires us to follow a DRESS Code. Longevity is as simple as optimizing each of the DRESS Code lifestyle elements, so we can live a healthier, longer life.

In this book, you will learn how to apply the DRESS Code to change the expression of your genes to optimize your health and longevity. Each chapter will provide concepts and practical tips for how to use these core elements in your life to achieve your health goals.

Based on my clinical experiences in caring for patients like Miguel and many others, unlocking the DRESS Code is the key that all of us need. Chronic conditions that make us sick, like diabetes, are not inevitable. We have the power to change this both as individuals and as a society. Instead of waiting until we are sick, we must address the root causes of illness by proactively focusing on prevention and lifestyle changes to promote health. In this way, we can use the core elements of the DRESS Code as guideposts to be healthier, feel younger, and live longer.

—Shad Marvasti, MD, MPH

PART I

Foundations
of the DRESS Code

CHAPTER 1

FROM "SICK" CARE TO "HEALTH" CARE

Why focus on *prevention* and *health* instead of *treatment* and *disease*? Before diving in each of the core elements of the DRESS Code, it's important to understand why prevention as part of a proactive approach to staying healthy throughout life is the key to combating the chronic diseases of our time. While treatment is critical, an ounce of prevention has always been worth more than a pound of cure. Waiting to get sick before you do something about it doesn't make sense.

For example, every day we put our lives at risk when we drive our cars. We don't wait until we have an accident and then hope for acute medical care to save our life. As individuals, we try to avoid accidents by learning how to drive properly, keeping distance between other cars, and wearing a seatbelt. As a society, we create traffic laws and signals to make it easier for us to be safe. Furthermore, our cars are designed with airbags and numerous safety features to prevent harm in the setting of an accident.

We can apply this approach to our health. Individually, we can avoid disease by how we live our life with a proper diet and balanced exercise and movement. As a society, we can make it easier to be healthy, just like traffic signals and laws help us avoid accidents. Unfortunately, not everyone obeys traffic laws, which results in too many motor vehicle accidents. In the same way, too many of us make poor choices for our health, and we get little guidance from most doctors on how to make better choices. And compared to the signals and traffic laws that help us stay safe on the road, our society sets us up to fail, with signals and incentives that make us prematurely sick.

Unlike in Blue Zones, where people live healthier for longer, in our society, people are living sicker for longer. It's no picnic just *technically* being alive into our eighties or nineties when we are debilitated or ill and unable to care for ourselves. I have seen this in many patients and in members of my own family. This is in large part due to a striking difference between a Blue Zone community and our society.

In the Blue Zones, the easy path of least resistance is the healthy path, making it possible for people to stay healthy for longer with little additional effort on their part. By comparison, in our society and in many parts of the developed world, the easy path is the unhealthy one. This default path is the path toward premature, preventable chronic disease.

When you have fast-food establishments all over the place and grocery stores loaded with processed foods, it's no wonder that so many, like Miguel and his family, are impacted by diabetes and obesity. When everyone drives, instead of walking or bicycling, we are less active, which makes us more prone to disease.

When we become socially isolated in our "garage" neighborhoods, where we don't know our neighbors and experience loneliness, we are at higher risk of illness and premature death. When the stress we feel is overwhelming all the time, we experience chronic inflammation that leads to chronic disease.

All these factors and more contribute to a world where getting a chronic disease is easy and staying healthy is difficult. Learning from places like the Blue Zones can make a huge difference in setting us up for success instead of failure.

The DRESS Code is a framework that includes all the key factors we need to live healthier for longer. But what about our healthcare system—is it at least helping to combat all these social, behavioral, and lifestyle determinants that are making us sick? Is it proactively teaching us how to stay healthy and empowering us to make good choices?

Sadly, the answer is no.

Our Sick Care System

We do not have a "healthcare" system. What we have is a reactive, acute disease management "sick care" system. As a postdoc at the Stanford Prevention Research Center (SPRC) in 2011, I wrote my vision statement for the revolution we needed in healthcare. This piece, coauthored with one of my faculty mentors, was accepted for publication in the *New England Journal of Medicine* as a perspective piece. It was aptly titled "From Sick Care to Health Care: Reengineering Prevention into the U.S. System."

In researching to write this article, I realized that our healthcare system allocates very little resources toward prevention. I also realized that the model of care we have is antiquated. This model was set up over a hundred years ago to combat the acute infectious diseases that were prevalent at the turn of the nineteenth century.

When our current system was set up in the early 1900s, chronic disease was uncommon. Most people were suffering and dying from acute infectious conditions like typhoid fever or tuberculosis. At that time, it made sense to focus on treatment rather than disease. It also made sense to buttress the bulwark of our public health system with sanitation systems and processes to prevent the spread of these infectious conditions.

However, as early as the 1930s, public health officials studying epidemiology noticed a shift away from acute conditions as we successfully knocked them out. While antibiotics and vaccines have received most of the credit for this massive decrease in acute infectious conditions, most of this occurred through public health and sanitation measures before the first antibiotic or vaccine was invented.

As time went on, acute diseases waned, and chronic disease took over. Despite the major shift in epidemiology, which now finds chronic disease as the major global cause of premature disease and death, medicine continues to operate under more than a century-old acute care model. Sadly, not much has changed since I published my paper arguing for a shift toward a prevention-focused model more than twelve years ago.

It's a difficult situation that most of us find ourselves in. With the path of least resistance being the path toward a chronic disease, most of us don't go to the doctor's office until we are sick. And once sick, we usually spend less than seven minutes with our doctor and go out the door with a medication. In fact, two-thirds of all doctor's visits in the United States result in a medication prescription. We rely on medications and surgery as a heroic measure to save lives in acute crisis.

Many, if not most, physicians work like first responders to treat people who are sick. Our entire system of insurance and reimbursement for care is set up for episodic, fee-for-service "sick" visits, where patients aren't seen until they are already ill with symptoms. We have a huge shortage of primary care physicians who can work with us over time to help us stay healthy.

When you do finally see your primary care doctor, you have very little time with them. Primary care doctors are literally running on a hamster wheel to go through as many patients as possible every day. With this frenetic pace, there is no time to discuss prevention, let alone empowering lifestyle practices to promote health and treat your medical condition naturally.

This perpetuates the need to see a high volume of patients without adequate time to focus on health and prevention. It also makes it easier simply to prescribe a medication as doctors are getting patients out the door. Even the documentation for clinical visits is focused on illness and disease. Medical students are taught that the first point they include in their documentation is the "Chief Complaint" followed by the "History of Present Illness," commonly referred to as the HPI. While acutely treating patients is critical and important in saving lives, waiting until people are sick before beginning to address their health sets both physicians and their patients up for failure and is not a good strategy for success.

Much of the burden of disease is now attributable to lifelong or chronic diseases. Chronic diseases are the leading cause of both disease and death worldwide. Seventy-one percent of all 56 million annual deaths worldwide are caused by chronic conditions.[2]

According to the CDC, the United States leads the world in chronic disease, where six in ten adults are living with a chronic disease, and four in ten are living with two or more chronic conditions. Seventy-five to eighty cents of every dollar spent on medical care in the United States is being spent on chronic diseases. Globally, heart disease, cancer, diabetes, and chronic lung diseases account for 80 percent of all chronic disease–related deaths.[3] In the United States, heart disease, cancer, and diabetes are now responsible for seven out of every ten deaths among Americans each year and account for up to 75 percent of the nation's health expenditures.

So, it's no mystery what the diseases of our time are. The question is, how can we prevent heart disease, or is it inevitable for us to get it? What about diabetes or cancer? Just like Miguel and his family, diabetes and other chronic conditions are not inevitable, nor are they a death sentence. The reality is that all three of these major diseases of our time are caused by modifiable risk factors and are therefore largely preventable—and in some cases even reversible.

Prevention Is Key

The word *prevention* comes from the Latin root, *praeventus*, to antici-pate or forestall from coming. The concept of disease prevention includes all efforts to anticipate the development of a disease and forestall it from developing and making us sick. Pushing disease later into our lifespan does not mean we will always cure it. So, the focus of prevention is not on waiting to cure us once we are sick. Instead, the focus of prevention is to push back the development of diseases like heart disease or cancer for as long as possible. While it is critical to have the best acute care possible when someone expe-riences a heart attack or stroke, the goal of prevention is to ensure this debilitating and life-threatening event does not happen in the first place.

Once you have a heart attack or stroke, your life may never be the same. Damage to your heart or brain can be permanent, leading to a long series of events that decrease your ability to live a full and enjoyable life. Here again, like driving, it is much bet-ter to prevent the accident from happening in the first place. For example, traffic signals prevent accidents, just like access to safe recreational facilities and parks can make it easy for us to exer-cise regularly to prevent high blood pressure, strokes, and heart attacks. Having inexpensive healthy foods can prevent us from becoming obese or developing a chronic disease. The opposite is sadly more common, and that's what makes disease prevention so critically important.

However, that being said, no disease can be prevented forever. Contrary to medicine's best efforts and intentions, we must accept the fact that eventually all of us will get sick and die. That much is inevitable. But *when* we get sick, and *how* we age is not inevitable. Otherwise, there would be no reason for you to read this book.

Fortunately, there is much you can do to help prevent you from getting sick in the first place. Both the timing of illness and its progression can be changed by our lifestyle. This is the key behind the DRESS Code. With it, we unlock our ability to live a younger, longer, and healthier life. The goal is not simply to live longer or expand our chronological lifespan. We want to expand our health-span. Healthspan—as opposed to lifespan—is the period of life when we can live fully without disease or disability. And therefore, the goal of prevention is to live *better* for longer. It's about experiencing health and wellness with a high quality of life for as long as possible. Being technically alive is not something any of us should strive for. Longevity is only great if those extra years are healthy years, as is the case in the Blue Zones, where people are not just surviving, but thriving to age one hundred.

Unsuccessful or unhealthy aging occurs when there is no emphasis on prevention. As chronic disease insidiously takes away from our ability to enjoy our lives, we see the consequences of simply allowing the aging process to accelerate without prevention or an investment in health. This is sadly how many of us age.

To understand what this aging looks like, let's look at functional capacity and how it changes over time. Functional capacity is the ability to perform daily activities at a high level with an exceptional quality of life. Most estimates of functional capacity show a significant and steady decline in several physiological systems as early as age forty-five. Decline accelerates after the first seminal event, like a heart attack or stroke, resulting in hospitalization. The resulting decline continues with decades of recurrent hospitalizations, admissions to rehabilitation centers, and ultimately, assisted living care facilities that together account for exorbitant costs and poor quality of life.

As bleak as this picture appears, aging experts have asserted that only 20 to 30 percent of the characteristics of aging are genetically based, and that environmental factors play a more critical role in the process. The science of epigenetics shows us that the social, behavioral, and lifestyle determinants of health are far more impactful than the genes we inherit at birth. Therefore, the evidence strongly supports the idea that we can do something about getting sick, making prevention a realistic and critical goal.

I have taken care of patients who are in nursing homes or home-bound with chronic illnesses that have debilitating symptoms, making these individuals unable to care for themselves. In far too many cases, I have seen people suffering from dementia who cause pain to their loved ones by not remembering who they are. Instead of working to prevent these tragedies, we accept them as inevitable. This is not life. This is not the goal of medicine or healthcare. While it is important to do our best to keep all these people alive, we can and must do better. Our goal with prevention is about quality, not quantity. The goal should be healthspan, not lifespan.

In contrast to the goal of expanding our healthspan, our current sick care system is a reactive, disease management system focused only on efficiencies in treatment, with little emphasis on prevention. While you want the state-of-the-art technology and medical science when you need immediate treatment for a heart attack or stroke, achieving optimal prevention means you won't have that life-changing event until much later (if ever)—toward the end of your life, rather than in middle age.

Another important concept is the nature of that heart attack or stroke. While acute conditions usually have a rapid onset and are self-limited in their disease course, chronic diseases have a gradual onset and are progressive over time. Acute conditions like the common cold usually come on quickly and resolve themselves in about a week. One does not "catch" a heart attack like a cold virus; rather, a heart attack is the acute exacerbation of the chronic process of atherosclerosis (the underlying process of narrowing and hardening of our arteries that results in heart disease).

Evidence of this comes from many sources, including atherosclerotic streaks found in Vietnam War veterans in their early to mid-twenties. As the disease process for acute and chronic diseases differs, so does their treatment. Acute disease usually involves supportive measures, such as in the case of the common cold, or targeted therapies for bacterial infections, such as strep throat.

On the other hand, chronic conditions such as type 2 diabetes require more complex treatment plans. And, due to their chronic nature, there is more time to intervene for longer periods before major health consequences arise. In the case of diabetes, these preventable consequences include blindness, kidney failure, lower limb amputation, and death. Thanks to the chronic nature of the disease, you have a larger window of opportunity to prevent its negative consequences if you act early.

This was the case for Miguel and for many patients like him whom I have had the privilege of treating in my medical practice. In order for the millions of people suffering from these chronic conditions to achieve relief, we must shift from an acute care reactive approach to a proactive long-term one that is focused on promoting health and prevention.

As individuals, we need to be proactive in our mindset and lifestyles about staying healthy, instead of waiting to get sick. And healthcare professionals must shift their focus from simply being a first responder as a doctor to being a coach who helps empower their patients with the tools they need to prevent disease in the first place. Sometimes this may be the physician, and other times, it may be a dietician or a health coach, who together form an interprofessional team that is able to support people as they make these healthy changes in their lives.

The significance of this shift and the value of primary prevention is best understood by the "River Story" or "Upstream Story" in public health. As the story goes, imagine a river with a high waterfall. At the bottom of the fall, there are hundreds of people who have fallen into the river and down the waterfall and are drowning. First responders and lifeguards are overwhelmed with so many people and are frantically working to rescue as many as they can.

These rescuers are like today's physicians, focused on acute care, constantly trying to save "drowning" patients from life-threatening conditions with heroic acts (high-tech, high-cost hospital-based medicine).

Continuing with the analogy, one person looks up and sees an endless stream of people falling down the waterfall. He goes upstream to see what is causing these people to fall. The others around him who are trying to save those who are drowning can't understand why this person isn't helping, instead of running upstream to find out what is going on. This is analogous to the need for us to shift from sick care to healthcare, from only treatment to primary prevention. It's moving away from simply applying Band-Aids with medications or surgeries for chronic conditions to addressing root causes by giving patients food and exercise prescriptions to prevent and reverse the causes of these conditions.

We need to practice what has been dubbed "Upstream Medicine" or "Upstream Healthcare" to address the root causes of the diseases of our time and prevent them from happening in the first place. By moving upstream, we can be proactive, instead of simply waiting until people are in a late-stage disease to receive heroic life-saving procedures. The time to act is always now—or even more accurately, yesterday. As the adage goes, "Do not put off till tomorrow what you can do today."

Back in 2011, my faculty mentor at Stanford, Dr. Randall Stafford, and I developed a graph to illustrate this concept. I went on to include this graph in a chapter I wrote in 2017 for a medical textbook on integrative preventive medicine. The common fate for many of us is unfortunately the red line where we are diagnosed with a chronic disease with a seminal event like a heart attack. This then results in a loss of our ability to live our life to the fullest or loss of our functional capacity. In this path we continue to decline getting sicker and sicker over time. Our current approach in medicine is reactive and focused on managing disease and not focused on keeping us healthy, so we end up with this first curve where we may still live longer but our healthspan is significantly decreased.

Functional Decline Over Time: Optimal DRESS vs Poor DRESS Code Lifestyle Elements

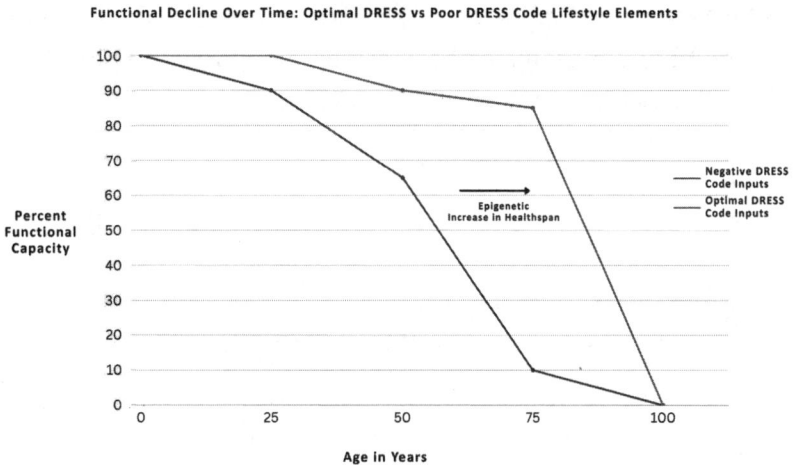

This graphic is an adaptation of a graph that was originally developed by Farshad Fani Marvasti (Shad Marvasti) and Randal S. Stafford and first published in "Integrative Preventive Medicine," Edited by Richard S. Carmona and Mark Liponis, in Chapter 6: The Role of Family and Community in Integrative Preventive Medicine written by Farshad Fani Marvasti, MD, MPH, ISBN 10: 019024125X ISBN 13: 9780190241254 Publisher: Oxford University Press, 2017.

Shifting this curve to the right with Optimal DRESS Code Lifestyle elements—Diet, Relationships, Exercise, Stress, and Sleep—that provide positive epigenetic inputs results in a longer healthspan and maintenance of our ability to live healthier for longer. Increasing healthspan by shifting the aging curve to the right is a win/win for everyone. Not only does this approach result in increased functional capacity and quality of life, but it also saves hundreds of billions of dollars that are currently being spent on care for the long period of illness that affects most of our population. By shifting the graph to the right through the delay of disease progression and illness onset, billions of dollars now spent on chronic disease management can be saved. In this way, we can improve the individual quality of life and simultaneously reduce the costs to our healthcare system. People can thrive to age one hundred like they do in the Blue Zones, instead of limping along for years in a tragic path toward senility and death.

CHAPTER 2

THERE IS NO LONGEVITY GENE: LIFESTYLE MATTERS MORE

Much has been written on long-lived people and centenarians, who seem to have effectively compressed morbidity and maximized their access to a high-quality disease-free life. These individuals do not live in a vacuum, but within a culture. The daily patterns, practices, and habits of these folks are reflected in their communities. They exist all over the world in areas popularly termed Blue Zones.

Exploration into these communities where healthspans have been maximized reveals several factors they have in common. These factors are not genetic in the strictest sense of the word. In other words, there is no Fountain of Youth in the form of a longevity gene that we can simply splice in or out of anyone to achieve this kind of life. Instead, it is a constellation of lifestyle factors, including dietary habits, physical activity levels, meaningful authentic relationships, and mental/emotional/spiritual beliefs and attitudes, which have a profound impact on our ability to compress morbidity and age well. In other words, the same advice that many of us received from our parents and grandparents about making friends, eating our "greens," and getting a good night's sleep are actually the key to health and longevity.

The opposite is also true. For example, isolation and sadness has been tied to immune function, health outcomes, and longevity. In dealing with the COVID-19 pandemic, many elderly family members were isolated to protect themselves from the virus, even though receiving hugs and physical touch from family would have boosted their immunity and helped them live better for longer. While this situation presents difficult-to-navigate challenges, what we do in terms of behavior and lifestyle throughout our lives determines how we are in our older years.

As it turns out, these social, behavioral, and lifestyle determinants of health are critically important. In fact, data shows that up to 40 percent of all cancers and 80 percent of premature heart disease, stroke, and diabetes can be prevented by addressing these critical risk factors.[4] If there was a medication that could do that, it would be the most prescribed medication on earth.

Going back to the "River Story" in the previous chapter, these determinants of health are the upstream causes of disease, the reasons people keep falling down the waterfall of disease and ultimately end up needing heroic medical care to save them from "drowning" to death. That's what I was dealing with as a medical resident with the seemingly endless cycle of patients with chronic conditions coming in and out, then back into the hospital through a revolving door of decline and illness. Thankfully, for the patients I have had the privilege of treating, like Miguel and his family, the upstream causes are factors that are ultimately in our control both as individuals and as a society. The practical steps to achieve this kind of lifelong wellness are reflected in the core elements of the DRESS Code. Before diving in further into each of these elements, let's first understand the scientific basis for the DRESS Code.

The Scientific Basis for the DRESS Code

At the molecular level, all life is linked to the repair and replication of deoxyribonucleic acid commonly referred to as DNA. Genetics is the study of inheritance patterns of DNA. The units of this inheritance are called genes, which are essentially our body's "software" packages that "code" who we are. Variations in genes and mutations contribute to our phenotype, which is the physical expression of our genes. Recognizing what genes contribute to what qualities, from simple features such as hair color to more complex features such as risk for a heart attack or stroke, has been a focus area of medicine since the discovery of DNA.

DNA includes the group of master molecules that are responsible for life at the molecular level. When we first discovered the role of DNA as the master molecule of life, scientists were excited about what this meant for medicine and the understanding of disease. What also emerged was the idea that everything was determined by our genes and that the only way to change things was to change our genes, which was impossible. This concept of genetic determinism basically concluded that some of us were "lucky" to inherit "good" genes that kept us healthy, while others were the unfortunate recipients of "bad" genes that made us sick.

With genetic determinism, control was taken out of our hands and given to our genes. This belief supported the notion that disease was caused by genes and could not be altered by our actions. For example, viewing alcoholism as a genetic disease where our choices don't matter, and we are doomed to have the same conditions that our parents had. In this worldview, we don't have a choice in why we get sick; it just happens to us because of the DNA that we have been hardwired with from birth, as it was passed down to us by our biological parents. The hope was that we would eventually be able to map out the entire genome, leading to the ability to edit out the bad genes and replace them with good ones that keep us healthy.

With the arrival of the Human Genome Project, our hopes were real-ized. In order to study the human genome, an Office for Human Genome Research was created at the National Institutes of Health in 1988. As someone who served as United States Surgeon General, I had the privilege of being involved with the public rollout of the Human Genome Project from 2002 to 2006. It was indeed humbling for me to meet Dr. James Watson, a Nobel laureate and co-discoverer of the double helix structure of DNA, as well as Dr. Craig Vetner, a former NIH genome scientist and visionary scientific innovator and entrepreneur. I also had the privilege of working closely with Drs. Francis Collins and Alan Guttmacher, the then-leaders of the National Human Genome Project. Our goal was to translate the rap-idly evolving genomic science in a health literate and culturally com-petent manner, so as to democratize this work for the public good. We excitedly poured resources into what we believed to be a new era of precision medicine focused on literally editing out bad genes through gene therapy. Despite the promise that the Human Genome Project would unlock human potential by enabling us to eliminate disease by identifying and eventually modifying our genes, we still are in the stages of infancy when it comes to applying this science to human health. The promise continues to be developed daily.

—Richard Carmona

While we wait to see when we may be able to modify genes in the future, something more exciting and immediately actionable has developed that challenges the concept of genetic determin-ism: the new science of epigenetics. With this new science, we now know that, save for a few genetically determined diseases, genetic determinism is *not* the cause of premature aging and the chronic diseases of our time. And even in the case of known genetic dis-eases, many of them can also be treated with improved outcomes based on how we live our life. The reason for this has to do with how our genes are turned "on" or "off" by the way we live and what we are exposed to.

While some genes are clearly "bad," resulting in certain degenerative diseases like Huntington's chorea, most genes are not clearly good or bad. Even specific physical traits like height are more complex than originally thought. These traits are not determined by single genes. Height, for example, is determined by more than twenty genes, the interactions of which researchers do not fully understand.

In looking at how genes contribute to disease, the picture is even more complicated. Most traits and conditions, including the most common chronic diseases of our time, like heart disease, diabetes, cancer, and obesity, are what we call polygenic diseases. These can be traced to combinations of "normal" genes. They are not the result of a single bad gene that can simply be edited out as previously believed. Instead, these conditions have multiple genetic sequences or snippets that combine in complex ways with our environment to increase or decrease our risk for disease. The interactions between these genes and the environmental inputs become more critical than the genes themselves. Of course, genes have a more pronounced role in certain rare genetic defects, like trisomy 21 or Tay-Sachs disease, but this is not the case for most people. Most of us are impacted by chronic conditions that arise from a society that is set up for us to get sick by making poor lifestyle choices, the easy choices to make.

The latest science has now proven that genes can be "turned on" or "turned off." As Dr. Ken Pelletier notes in his groundbreaking book *Change Your Genes, Change Your Life*, our epigenome "responds to how we interact with our world."[5]

Epi literally means "above or upon which." The term *epigenetics* is the "science of that which is above and beyond the gene." So, what is beyond the gene? Aren't genes the master molecules of life? Yes. And genes can't be edited or changed as hoped by the

Human Genome Project? Well, the answer to that is yes and no. Genes themselves cannot be changed, but they can be turned on or off; their expression can be changed. Gene expression can change in response to how we interact with the world. Our genes' response includes what genes are expressed, essentially being turned on or off by our environmental and behavioral inputs—e.g., how we live our life. This happens at an epigenetic level, above and beyond the genes themselves. It occurs through complex inputs and interactions with our environment—how we eat, sleep, exercise, think, and act.

The core elements of the DRESS Code are all epigenetic inputs. The resulting new paradigm that emerges is similar to the cloud concept for the internet, where a complex web of interactions between our genes, actions, and beliefs determines if, when, and how we get sick. This is the new model of medicine that is more accurate and effective as we charge into artificial intelligence and other emerging technologies. It emphasizes the importance of lifestyle and provides evidence for how this changes us at the molecular level, at the level of our genes.

The best way to understand how changing gene expression impacts our health is by appreciating a computer analogy for our genes. Genes are the software, and our bodies are the hardware. Genes are the operating system for how life is born, grows, develops, and functions throughout the lifespan. Just like your computer's operating system can be updated, so too, can the genes that run our lives. The way genes update their versions is through their gene expression, and these changes are above and beyond the genes themselves, making them epigenetic.

If we think of our genes as software packages, we get to write and re-write that software code every day by how we choose to live and what we are exposed to in life. A bad gene that is not expressed does not cause harm. While a good gene that is expressed can prevent harm. Epigenetics, or that which is above or beyond the genes, is the software, the environmental inputs (how we live our life) that determine what genes are used and what genes remain dormant. The software determines the outcome. You need the hardware, but it's the software that is key to determining what you look like and how well you operate. We need our genes to get the basic elements of development in life, but it is how we live that determines how sick or healthy we become. Good software can make the best of bad hardware, while good hardware can be trashed by bad software. If you have a clunky software system, like a poor diet, the best engineered computer system will perform poorly, with delays and glitches.

The same is true of our bodies. How we choose to live in the core elements of the DRESS Code can provide the best epigenetic inputs that allow us to live healthier for longer. How we live can also provide negative epigenetic inputs that make matters worse, leading to premature disease and death. For example, if we have great genetics, but we insist on eating processed foods, being inactive without enough sleep, and are subject to chronic unhealthy stress in life, then we will age prematurely and have a shorter healthspan despite the good genes we inherit at birth. If, on the other hand, we eat real, nutrient-dense foods and find ways to cope with stress, building resilience and a sense of purpose, we will enjoy a longer, healthier life.

One of the best sources of evidence of the power of epigenetics to impact our health is found in research studies of identical twins. Identical twins have identical—or the same—DNA down to every base nucleotide pair. There is no genetic difference between them. While the underlying DNA does not change over time in identical twins, twin studies have shown that the epigenome or the expression of these genes changes and varies significantly over time in different ways for each twin. The epigenome determines what genes are expressed, when they are expressed, and how they are expressed. In these now-famous twin studies, we know that the conditions under which these twins lived determined their health and life outcomes. These conditions included lifestyle choices, such as what they ate, how active they were, and the level of stress in their lives. These social, behavioral, and lifestyle determinants of health explained the changes in their epigenome or genetic software over time.

So, while the DNA provides the raw hardware for life and can be faulty in certain rarer conditions, the software is written by us with our daily decisions. We provide the code by messaging our genes to turn on and off by what we eat, how we act, and what we believe. Instead of being doomed to becoming sick because of our genetic code, we can change the course of our lives with the DRESS Code. Thus, the answers to why we get sick and what we can do are unlocked by how we live our life, which is the essence of the DRESS Code.

Biohacking 101 and the DRESS Code

A popular term among many health and wellness enthusiasts for preventing sickness and stopping aging in its tracks is *biohacking*. Biohacking represents an innovative approach to do it yourself (DIY) for optimizing health and longevity. Biohacking is about engaging in activities and practices to change our chemistry and physiology through science-inspired techniques. Biohacking involves systematic changes to our lifestyle, like intermittent fasting, which when done correctly, can reverse aging and enhance our ability to stay healthy. It's based on the idea that we are not destined by our genes to be sick. Rather, we can hack our system to optimize our health. Based on the new science of epigenetics, I believe that biohacking is justifiably popular because when done right, it can work wonders. The DRESS Code is essentially the ultimate DIY biohacking toolkit to unlock our greatest potential for optimal health and longevity.

Biohackers have realized that our current approach to medicine is severely limited by focusing too narrowly on disease treatment instead of prevention and health. That's why many seek and pay for biohacking solutions outside the current medical system. The problem is that too often people are confused by the numerous options available to them. Some biohackers advocate for a keto-genic diet and intermittent fasting, while others choose to focus on a completely plant-based vegan diet. Still others talk about a hybrid diet called paleo or pegan. Millions of people flock to their favorite biohacker for tips on how to unlock and "hack" their system to achieve health. While some of these biohacking strategies are based in science, others are potentially harmful or have no effect at all, thus costing us money and time.

My goal with the DRESS Code is to distill the latest scientific evidence, along with my clinical experiences in caring for patients, to give you the best DIY biohacking toolkit available. The DRESS Code is based on the science of epigenetics. I have witnessed how changing your lifestyle can change your life by fundamentally changing you at the level of your DNA.

With the DRESS Code, I have identified what works, what is potentially harmful, and why. I will also explain why a "one size fits all" approach (with some exceptions) does not work for every-one. Some have proposed that this personalized approach should be based on our unique genetic or molecular profile. The use of this profile to optimize medicine is known as *precision health*. Much research is now being focused on tailoring treatments, such as medications and medication dosages, to our genetic profile. For example, our genetic differences determine how quickly our body metabolizes or breaks down a given drug. Generally speaking, the faster you metabolize a medication, the higher dose you may need. Identifying whether you are a slow, intermediate, or fast metabo-lizer for a class of medications can be a useful tool in dosing medi-cations appropriately.

However, as useful as genetic profiling and precision medicine can potentially be, it's not as impactful as optimizing epigenetic inputs. That's why I prefer to shift the focus in this book from precision medicine to precision health. By focusing on precision health, I want to empower you to discover your own personalized approach that's designed to work for you based on applying the DRESS Code to your life. I want you to learn what works for you. This can be both revolutionary and safe. Much of what I will cover in this book is essentially a DIY guide to biohacking. This includes debunking myths and providing key insights into diet, exercise, and lifestyle that are based on the best available, most innovative scientific evidence of our time.

I hope that in learning about the DRESS Code, you'll be able to have an informed conversation with your healthcare provider to prevent or even reverse disease before it's too late. We will delve deeper into each part of this biohacking puzzle to share the best practices and practical steps that you need to begin working on things today to impact your health tomorrow and well into the future.

Throughout this book, I will explain how epigenetic inputs act like software to code for health or disease, depending on our choices. Remember, the DRESS Code is based on the fact that our choices change gene expression. The epigenetic tags formed by our lifestyle choices are even passed on to the next generation. So, our choices impact not only us but can impact the health of our children at the molecular level. The stakes couldn't be higher. The DRESS Code is based on the science of epigenetics to give meaning to the wisdom passed on from generations of abuelas (grandmothers) and family members to teach us how to live our best life. These practices, such as home remedies and folk medicine, have been with us for thousands of years across the globe. With the new science, we can now see how and why these practices have worked well to keep people living healthier for longer in places like the Blue Zones. The DRESS Code puts it all together in an easy-to-understand and practical approach to why we should exercise, eat healthy, and address the social determinants of health.

Remember, software beats hardware every time. Without getting the software right, the hardware is no good to you. In fact, bad software can lead to a poorly functioning system that in turn leads to premature loss of function. When applied to the human body, this means premature, unhealthy aging. For example, the fact that processed food currently makes up greater than 60 percent of the Standard American Diet (SAD) is an example of bad software that epigenetically interferes with our hardware or bodies to make us sick. Living an inactive or sedentary lifestyle without any physical activity is another example of bad inputs leading to negative outputs from the expression of disease-causing genes.

Like new software upgrading a computer, our choices to live a healthy lifestyle can reprogram (or recode) our genes to help us live healthier for longer and achieve the goal of prevention. Like any software update, applying the DRESS Code to your life will make your hardware run smoother. It's made up of simple, practical steps you can take to upgrade your life.

Who you are at birth is largely determined by the genetic information passed on to you by your parents. But who you will be in life is largely determined by your health behaviors and the choices you make to upgrade or downgrade your genes throughout your life. By unlocking the DRESS Code, you can code for health, wellness, and longevity instead of disease, premature aging, and early death. Think of the DRESS Code as a blueprint for your life, mapping out the key points and patterns of healthy habits that you need to expand your healthspan and stay well for as long as possible.

CHAPTER 3

THE DISEASES OF OUR TIME AND THEIR ROOT CAUSES

Each of the core DRESS Code elements impacts our health in a variety of ways. Each of these elements can increase or decrease chronic inflammation. Chronic inflammation is at the root of each of the major chronic diseases of our time. It impacts us in a variety of ways and also relates to the epigenetic changes that occur based on how we live our life. The complex interactions between our lifestyle, inflammation, and epigenetic changes make up the fundamental stuff of aging. Understanding this science is foundational to learning how to use the DRESS Code elements to slow down aging and increase our healthspan.

Two Kinds of Inflammation: Acute and Chronic

Inflammation is a part of life and is, in fact, a critical part of healing. A protective reaction to injury, disease, or irritation, inflammation can be, on occasion, lifesaving. But the protective part only applies to *acute inflammation*. It does not apply to long-term or *chronic inflammation*, which is the root cause of the diseases of our time.

Acute inflammation is part of the body's innate ability to heal itself in response to an injury from trauma or an invading pathogen (e.g., a harmful virus or bacterial species or even a toxic substance).

Acute inflammation comes on rapidly and usually lasts several hours or several days. All of us have experienced acute inflammation at some point. When you twist your ankle, cut yourself, or are bitten by a mosquito, these injuries result in an acute inflammatory response. You will usually experience a combination of several symptoms at the site of the injury, including redness, warmth, swelling, and pain. The redness, warmth, and swelling come from increased blood flow to the area to bring immune and repair cells to the site to address the injury. Pain is a signal that tells us to be careful in that spot and to stop and take it easy while our body takes the time it needs to heal the injury.

When we are infected with a virus, such as a cold or flu, we have a similar acute inflammatory response. For example, we may experience a rise in body temperature commonly known as a fever. A fever is an inflammatory response that makes it more difficult for the source of an infection like a virus to survive. Fevers thus provide us with an edge to mount our own immune response. We may experience internal swelling leading to mucous formation, which creates a barrier to stop the virus from spreading further. All these symptoms are part of the body's acute inflammatory response, which is essentially a healing response.

Studies have shown that, within a range of acceptable symptoms, it's best not to treat a fever or immediately reach for anti-inflammatory medication like ibuprofen, as that can thwart the immune response to the acute injury. One example of a fever that is helpful occurs after we receive a vaccine. After receiving a vaccine, our body begins to mount an immune response to the vaccine elements, which sometimes results in a fever. In this case, the acute inflammation is good, as our body is creating antibodies to build immunity against the virus we have been vaccinated for. Therefore, in these instances, we should avoid anti-inflammatory medications like ibuprofen, because using them will not allow our body to create protective antibodies. In these and other situations, while it may be helpful to seek relief from pain if it becomes unbearable, or a fever persists or is too high, it is important to recognize that pain and fever are a part of the natural healing response.

While acute inflammation is a healthy response to acute injury, chronic inflammation can be deadly. Chronic inflammation is slower in its onset than acute inflammation. It lasts longer, from as little as several months to many years. Usually, the initial cause may be similar to acute inflammation, but the "injury" involved is recurring, lower grade, and persistent over time. This is unlike what we experience after an acute injury, which is acute inflammation with high-grade symptoms. Chronic inflammation is low-grade, like a slow burn that gradually burns us away. This is the type of inflammation that is at the root of the chronic diseases of our time.

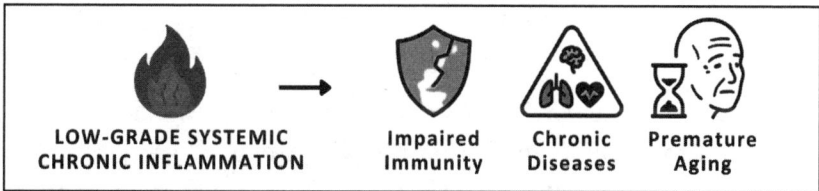

LOW-GRADE SYSTEMIC CHRONIC INFLAMMATION → **Impaired Immunity** · **Chronic Diseases** · **Premature Aging**

What Triggers Low-Grade Chronic Inflammation?

Understanding the causes of chronic inflammation is critical to recognizing the source of premature aging and premature disease. Some have described this chronic debilitating process as "inflammaging." This chronic inflammation that ages us is found as a core component of all the major chronic diseases of our time. Thankfully, the primary causes of chronic inflammation are not genetically determined and unchangeable. What we are exposed to and how we live our life are the strongest contributors to whether we have chronic inflammation or not. These are also the key epigenetic inputs that change the expression of our genes for better or for worse. Therefore, it is the exposome—the social, behavioral, and lifestyle determinants of health—that creates the main triggers for chronic inflammation and gene expression. Rather than something that is genetically predetermined, these factors are within our control. These triggers include a poor diet, unhealthy relationships or social isolation, a lack of physical exercise, chronic stress, and poor or disturbed sleep.

Chronic inflammation ultimately leads to premature disease, aging, and death. When we optimize these factors, we can prevent disease, expand our healthspan, and achieve longevity. For example, our diet can be either pro-inflammatory or anti-inflammatory. What we eat can contribute directly to chronic inflammation, or it can reduce it. The same is true for exercise, relationships, sleep, and the management of stress in our lives. These factors form the core elements of the DRESS Code: **D**iet, **R**elationships, **E**xercise, **S**tress, and **S**leep.

Diet

There are many examples that demonstrate how these factors can promote chronic inflammation. Eating processed food—or "Frankenfoods," as we like to call them—generate free radicals. Free radicals are reactive oxygen molecules that oxidize or damage aspects of the body, leading to chronic inflammation. This accumulation of free radicals and the resulting inflammation is a direct cause of premature aging. For example, when the free radicals generated by trans fats or hydrogenated oils (usually found in processed foods and industrially produced seed oils) damage low-density lipoprotein (LDL) cholesterol (the form of "bad" cholesterol linked to heart disease), the damaged LDL elicits an inflammatory response. This response leads to a cascade of chronic inflammation, which is the underlying process of atherosclerosis (narrowing of the arteries). This form of chronic inflammation ultimately leads to a heart attack or stroke.

Specific foods in excess can also be inflammatory. For example, excessive amounts of meat and seafood products can lead to high levels of uric acid and result in an acute gout attack. Higher uric acid is also a contributor to high blood pressure, which is a risk factor for a heart attack or stroke. Excess sodium can directly impair our immune systems and also increase our blood pressure, which increases our risk for both strokes and heart attacks. High-sugar diets and processed foods can cause diabetes and increase our risk for various kinds of cancer, as well as autoimmune conditions such as rheumatoid arthritis and lupus, where the immune system goes haywire by attacking healthy tissue. This is often triggered by gluten, lactose, or chemical additives in processed foods.

Relationships

Human beings are social creatures. Our relationships are not just a nice thing to have, but these, in fact, are critical for our health. Authentic, meaningful relationships have been shown to reduce chronic inflammation and increase our healthspan by improving risk factors for diseases like high blood pressure. Being connected with others, including physical touch, releases hormones like oxytocin that make us happy and reduce inflammation throughout our bodies. Having strong social ties has been identified as a key feature of the Blue Zones, where people live longer and healthier. Social support groups for diseases like cancer have been independently associated with longer lives and better health outcomes for people impacted by this life-threatening condition. Belonging to a group or community is a protective factor for both disease and death.

On the flip side, experiencing loneliness is associated with an increased risk for both premature disease and death. Some studies have even found the impact of loneliness to be on par with cigarette smoking. Social isolation contributes to anxiety and will increase chronic inflammation over time. This is a major contributor to chronic inflammation in our world, where we are virtually "connected" to streaming services and social media, only to find a lack of real connections that impact both our mental and physical health.

Exercise

Exercise, movement, and any physical activity reduce chronic inflammation and its ill effects. The lack of moving naturally throughout the day is responsible for many premature deaths, as it increases our risk for the chronic diseases of our time, including heart disease, diabetes, obesity, and cancer. Lack of physical activity, such as a cardio or aerobic exercise, where your pulse rate is elevated, is also a key factor in the development of dementia, as the aging brain needs higher oxygen levels and reduced inflammation provided by exercise to thrive.

Without physical activity, our muscles atrophy and contribute to a process known as sarcopenia or muscle wasting. Losing muscle mass is the single best predictor of premature aging, as it increases our risk of both disease and death. Exercise clears out inflammation, so inactivity maintains it and allows the fire of chronic inflammation to persist unchecked. In our modern world, sitting for long periods of time has been likened to smoking in some research where it has been shown to be an independent risk factor for chronic inflammation, leading to premature disease and death.

Stress

Stress can be good or bad. Chronic stress is unhealthy for the body and is the key source of chronic inflammation. While short-term stress like an ice bath, hot sauna, or vigorous exercise reduces inflammation, chronic stress—whether it be emotional or physical—is associated with the release of inflammatory cytokines (chemical messenger signals that go between cells). These chemicals lead to higher rates of inflammation over time. Chronic stress is multifaceted. This stress can come from a variety of social situations, from dealing with difficult relationships to financial problems, as well as how we perceive the world around us.

Even the microaggressions experienced by victims of discrimination can be a source of chronic inflammation. Both perceived discrimination and the reality of racism result in the increased production of cytokines, which increase inflammation and are major sources of chronic stress and chronic inflammation. This may explain why Black men have the highest rates of high blood pressure in America. We will explore the impact of this and other triggers in the chapter on stress.

Sleep

Sleep disorders cause their own kind of stress, so they are an independent risk factor for chronic inflammation. Sleep is a special activity that allows the body time and space to regenerate and reduce inflammation in every organ and tissue. It's not only the hours of sleep, but the quality of sleep that matters. In particular, it is important to maintain a certain number of "deep sleep" hours that begin to decline as we age. Sleep as part of a daily cycle is a key part of having predictability in patterns that contribute to health.

Lack of sleep is one of the most underrated and prevalent problems in the United States and around the world. Both inadequate hours of sleep and sleep quality are directly linked to an increase in markers of inflammation. Over time, this contributes to chronic inflammation, leading to a higher risk of high blood pressure, impaired immunity, disrupted hormonal patterns, and premature disease. The inflammation from lack of sleep also increases our risk for several cancers and dementia.

Connecting Epigenetics and Chronic Inflammation

The bad news is that any of the core DRESS Code elements can be potential triggers for inflammation. But the good news is that this also means they can be powerful tools to reduce inflammation, and now we can understand a more complex dynamic between these key factors: the state of inflammation in our bodies and the science of epigenetics.

The consequences of slow-burning, low-grade chronic inflammation ultimately include the most significant diseases and causes of premature death. Low-grade systemic chronic inflammation (SCI) has also been directly linked with premature aging at the cellular level, where our cells age at a more rapid rate. Over time, this chronic inflammation also impairs our immune function, which increases our risk for infections and tumors. Chronic inflammation leads to a plethora of unwanted results, such as:

- heart disease
- diabetes
- metabolic syndrome
- non-alcoholic fatty liver disease
- depression
- obesity
- autoimmune diseases
- neurodegenerative diseases (Alzheimer's, dementia)
- osteoporosis and muscle wasting
- cancer

These chronic conditions are caused by triggers that lead to chronic inflammation. Once these diseases take root, chronic inflammation increases. For example, people with diabetes who have uncontrolled blood sugar levels form advanced glycation end products (AGEs). AGEs are compounds in the bloodstream formed from damage that occurs to structures from excess glucose "bumping" into them. These damaged compounds elicit an inflammatory response that persists for as long as these continue to be formed. All this further contributes to the chronic inflammatory state.

Evidence is now emerging that the epigenetic processes that affect gene expression are key contributors to the chronic inflammation involved in these medical conditions. This leads to premature damage at the cellular, tissue, and organ levels. To put it simply, the changes that occur in gene expression can result in persistent inflammatory responses at the cellular and molecular levels.

The cell-to-cell changes of a persistent inflammatory response have been identified in the form of cytokines (chemical messengers between cells). Epigenetic changes have been linked to the development of some of the most well-known and well-researched pro-inflammatory cytokines that are involved in a variety of diseases, including but not limited to, many kinds of cancer, heart disease, diabetes, and neurodegenerative conditions.

The change in gene expression resulting from epigenetic inputs like diet or exercise is known as an *epigenetic signature*. Epigenetic signatures regulate the development of pro-inflammatory molecular pathways leading to the diseases of our time. For example, high consumption of simple sugars in the form of juice that is high in fructose has been linked to epigenetic signatures resulting in chronic inflammation. Another example is trans fat, a damaged, "bad" form of fat that has been implicated in heart disease. Eating foods with trans fat (or forming these by heating oil past the smoke point) changes gene expression and "downgrades" our genetic software, resulting in inflammation. This chronic inflammation, in turn, triggers the process of atherosclerosis, or the narrowing of our arteries through scarring and plaque formation. Over time, continued consumption of processed foods high in bad fats will ultimately increase our risk for heart attack or stroke.

On the other hand, omega 3 fatty acids have the opposite effect. Eating foods rich in these good fats, such as wild salmon or walnuts or ground flaxseed, "upgrades" our genetic software, offering a protective anti-inflammatory effect on our heart and blood vessels. Consuming food sources rich in monounsaturated fats (avocados, extra-virgin cold-pressed olive oil, pecans, and almonds) have been shown to have the same benefits and links to epigenetic changes that reduce inflammation. While many complex factors are involved, let's briefly discuss the most common genetic mechanisms to understand how the way we live can change our genes for the better.

The Importance of DNA Methylation, Histone Modification, and miRNA Regulation

Beneath the surface of the daily epigenetic inputs that determine our health and longevity are a complex series of molecular interactions between the genome (our genes) and exposome (our environment, including our lifestyle).

At the molecular level, epigenetics includes a group of chemical modifications of the DNA sequence directly affected by external epigenetic inputs—that is, the core elements of the DRESS Code. These core inputs can be either pro-inflammatory or anti-inflammatory. If inflammatory and persistent over time, the resulting chronic inflammatory molecules exert negative epigenetic changes on gene expression. In fact, research shows clear associations between DNA methylation and markers of inflammation in our blood. As previously noted, epigenetic modifications of DNA leading to changes in gene expression are dynamic and reversible through our lifestyle choices.

Epigenetics is the study of changes in gene expression, also known as cellular *phenotype*. Genotype refers to our genes—your genotype is your genetic makeup. Phenotype is the physical expression and outcome of what our genes or genotype codes for. Therefore, our genotype encodes our phenotype. For example, a combination of our genes (genotype) determines our height or eye color (phenotype). Except for rarer cases of genetically determined disease, how our genes interact with the environment is much more critical than any given gene. Remember the software analogy? As with software, our genes can be upgraded or downgraded depending on what we choose to adapt or take on in our lives. Therefore, the expression of our genes is regulated by what we do and how we live. Epigenetics examines how changes in gene expression can occur by mechanisms other than changes to the underlying DNA sequence. These mechanisms can include one or more combined elements of the DRESS Code that can upgrade our genetic software. These complex changes occur at the molecular level and include several key processes. We will focus on three major mechanisms:

- DNA methylation
- Histone modification
- miRNA regulation

DNA Methylation

DNA methylation is simply when a chemical structure known as a methyl group is potentially added to two of the DNA building blocks known as a nucleotide. You may have read about the chemical structure of DNA if you have taken a biology class or watched *Jurassic Park*. The four nucleotides (chemical structures) that form the backbone of the DNA double helix are adenine, cytosine, guanine, and thymine. Adenine and cytosine are the two that can be methylated as the result of lifestyle changes or epigenetic inputs. This is one mechanism for epigenetics.

Histone Modification

A second major mechanism for epigenetics is histone protein modification. Histone proteins are the chain that the DNA double helix winds around at the molecular level. Histone proteins can directly activate or repress gene expression. Histone proteins can also be modified by the DRESS Code epigenetic inputs.

miRNA Regulation

A third major mechanism is micro-ribonucleic acid (miRNA) regulation. These molecules surround the double helix of DNA and histone proteins, exerting another level of influence on gene expression. These molecules are directly impacted by the food we eat and the way we live. For example, research on resveratrol, an antioxidant found in grapes and berries, directly modifies the expression of a group of miRNA molecules involved in the regulation of the inflammatory response to high blood pressure. This may be one of the mechanisms for the heart health benefits of consuming resveratrol-rich foods, such as blueberries, grapes, and pomegranates.

The following diagram illustrates how epigenetic inputs result in changes to histone protein modification, DNA methylation, or micro-RNA (miRNA), which ultimately lead to changes in health outcomes, either positive or negative. The DRESS Code inputs optimize this process, leading to optimal health outcomes and longevity.

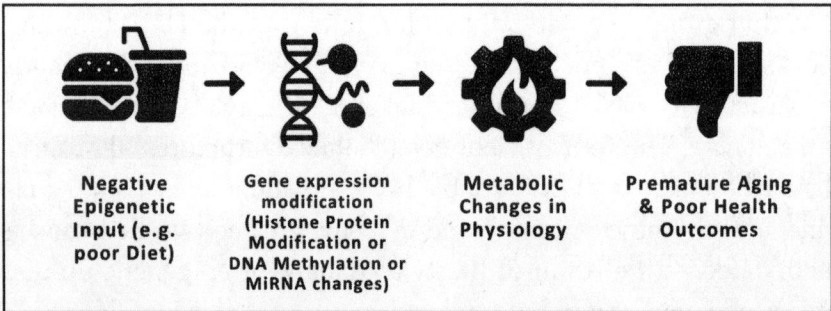

| Negative Epigenetic Input (e.g. poor Diet) | → | Gene expression modification (Histone Protein Modification or DNA Methylation or MiRNA changes) | → | Metabolic Changes in Physiology | → | Premature Aging & Poor Health Outcomes |

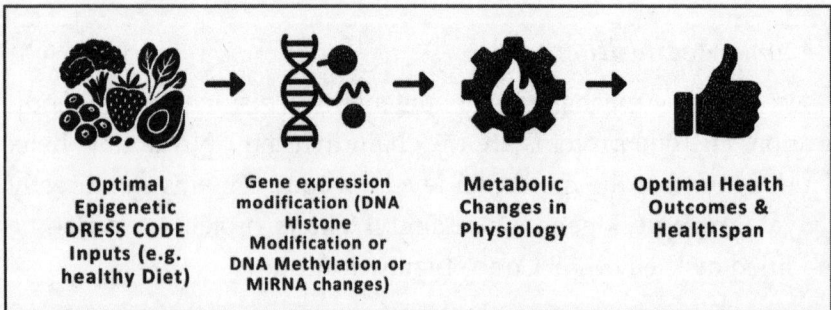

| Optimal Epigenetic DRESS CODE Inputs (e.g. healthy Diet) | → | Gene expression modification (DNA Histone Modification or DNA Methylation or MiRNA changes) | → | Metabolic Changes in Physiology | → | Optimal Health Outcomes & Healthspan |

Based on the science of epigenetics, the critical role that social, behavioral, and lifestyle determinants of health plays are obvious. This is the basis for the DRESS Code, along with the recognition that the source of life-shortening, deadly chronic inflammation is lifestyle. How we live our lives can change our genes and our fate, for better or worse. So, while the key DRESS Code elements can trigger chronic inflammation, they are also the cause of changes in our genetic software.

The good news is these elements can be changed for the better. We can reduce stress; we can alter our diet to change our genes and reduce inflammation. We can engage in anti-inflammatory activities that ensure we keep levels of chronic inflammation as low as possible while also optimizing our genetic software for health. Albeit more difficult and involved, we can also modify the social determinants of health by addressing health inequality and systemic structural racism by recognizing it as a public health crisis and dismantling the institutional elements that support it. We can strive to reform health policies and transform our communities to parallel Blue Zones where the easy path is the healthy path for more of us.

In the next several chapters, we explore exactly how we can target epigenetic inputs with each element of the DRESS Code to stimulate changes in gene expression to reduce inflammation and expand our healthspan.

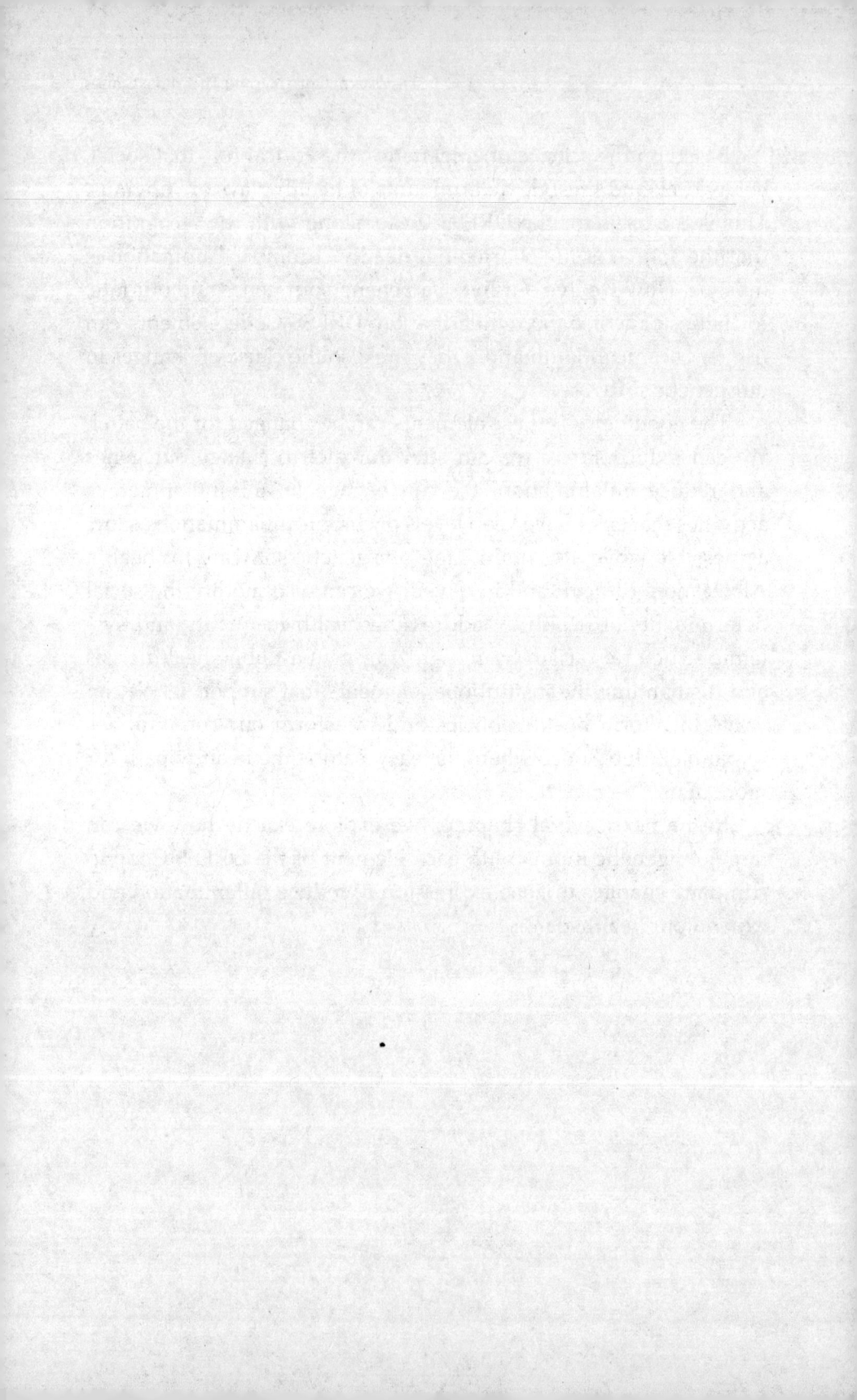

PART II

The DRESS Code

CHAPTER 4

D IS FOR DIET: EAT TO OPTIMIZE HEALTH

The Dress Code starts with D for diet. Diet is a major epigenetic input—which means that, at the molecular level, food can directly turn your genes on or off, thereby causing or curing disease with every bite you take. Food can upgrade your genetic software or downgrade it, leading to premature illness and death. Understanding food as an epigenetic input means there are both foods that heal you and foods that make you sick.

While the science of epigenetics is new, the concept of food as medicine is ancient. It's a concept that has spanned all parts of the globe over the last several thousand years. Over time, many cultures came to understand the importance of food as medicine by developing rituals and practices that honored and applied insights about food to their daily lives. Early physicians would often prescribe a dietary regimen as the cornerstone of their treatments. Healers or medicine men or women would tell their patients to stop this or add more of that, brew this tea or mix these herbs and vegetables together. All sorts of combinations would be tried to treat disease and preserve health.

In addition to folk medicine and family traditions for using food as part of home remedies, some cultures even developed entire medicinal systems around the proper amounts, mixtures, and preparations of food to stay healthy and treat illnesses. Some of these cultures, including those of China and India, are notable for the expansive body of knowledge and detailed classifications of foods they developed. These health systems, including Traditional Chinese Medicine (TCM) and Ayurvedic medicine, have mapped out patterns of health and illness and connected them with food.

Take, for example, Ayurvedic medicine, which developed in ancient India alongside Hinduism and is still practiced today. In this system, models were developed to classify individual personality types—known as doshas—that are prone to specific patterns of illness and require certain types of diets to keep them balanced. According to Ayurvedic medicine, some personality types benefit greatly from spicy foods to keep them alert and energetic, while others simply respond with too much "heat" from these foods, leading to irritability, anger, and increased susceptibility to disease. Ayurvedic practitioners argue that balancing our food choices results in balancing our personality and physiological tendencies, leading to health and well-being.

Similar approaches were also developed in China. In one of the main forms of TCM, foods are classified as warm/hot or cool/cold in nature, paralleling the concepts of yin and yang, which are loosely understood in analogies to be night and day or shadow and sun. Practitioners believe that balancing hot and cold foods is essential to preventing and treating disease that results from internal imbalances in the organs (which are also classified as naturally yin or yang).

While these long-standing empiric traditions, based on trial and error, have been passed down through generations of practitioners and families, modern science is now beginning to validate their dietary prescriptions and herbal remedies. Some of the major herbs and medicinal foods used in these health systems have been extensively researched and found to have many health benefits, including modifying specific diseases at the molecular level.

Some examples include garlic, ginger, and turmeric. The "active ingredient" in garlic, responsible for its pungent smell, has been found to have strong antimicrobial properties as well as antioxidant activity. Phytochemicals like curcumin in turmeric has been found to directly inhibit literally hundreds of molecular pathways leading to cancer and heart disease. Although evidence is mounting in these areas, therapeutic use of food is still not actively incorporated into mainstream conventional medicine (also known as *allopathic medicine*).

Conventionally trained doctors who undertake additional fellowship training in integrative medicine, certification in lifestyle medicine, functional medicine, or culinary medicine (more about these fields in Chapter 12) learn how to use food as medicine with targeted dietary therapies; however, the majority of conventional medical education and practice does not include nutrition or the precise use of food as medicine. Currently, using food as medicine is most passionately championed by biohackers and wellness experts, while most physicians (save for those in the fields mentioned above) remain unengaged in this area.

Instead, conventional Western medicine focuses on using medications and interventional or surgical procedures as their primary therapeutic tools. While medications are lifesaving, they do not come without costs, both in terms of potentially dangerous side effects and economic harms.

According to data compiled in several studies and the Food and Drug Administration, adverse drug reactions (ADRs) are the fourth leading cause of death, including cases when drugs were prescribed correctly with known side effects, deadly drug interactions, and dosing errors. And every surgery, while potentially lifesaving, comes with the risk of severe bleeding, infection, or death. Both surgery and medication can be powerful tools, but they are not always the best tools we have to stay healthy or treat contemporary diseases, because their potential to do harm is not insignificant. Diet as therapy definitely has less potential to do harm.

Now, the question arises: Is there enough evidence for nutrition to be a primary therapy—especially since it has less potential to do harm than both medications and surgery? And, if there is substantial evidence for it (which there is), why are doctors not using it more as the primary therapeutic option for their patients?

As our understanding of epigenetics grows through new research, we can see real examples of how diet continually updates our genetic software, programming us for health or disease depending on what we choose to eat. So, again, why is this option not a mainstay of medical treatment and prevention? The answer has less to do with the evidence for nutrition's role in health, and more to do with the fact that physicians are simply not trained in this critical epigenetic therapy.

Have you ever asked your doctor for advice on what to eat? In my experience, patients often get varied answers from most doctors that are either too general and inadequate or sometimes inaccurate. Some of my patients do get good advice from doctors they've visited in the past, but, by and large, most physicians have little knowledge or understanding of nutrition, which limits their ability to guide patients on what and when to eat. Most respond with generic answers like "Eat healthy" or "Eat less" without targeted dietary recommendations. Responses vary from "It doesn't really matter as long as you have good genes" to "Just make sure to take this medication and you don't have to worry about what you eat." Both responses are wrong.

So, why don't most doctors know more about nutrition? On average, in the United States, over four years of medical school, most medical students only get a total of 19.6 hours of nutrition education across all four years, according to a national survey.[6] Not 19.6 credit hours, but literally less than twenty hours of nutrition education. Recent surveys have shown that 71 percent of US medical schools fail to provide the recommended minimum twenty-five hours of nutrition education, and 36 percent provide less than half that much.[7]

Sadly, global systematic reviews have shown a similar trend, regardless of country. These deficits contribute to low levels of nutrition knowledge and confidence to counsel patients on nutrition in clinical practice. It's no wonder so many physicians think that, compared to all the other scientific facts and risk factors for disease and death, nutrition plays a relatively minor role. Sadly, nothing could be further from the truth.

Culinary Medicine

Culinary medicine is an innovation in medical education that bridges the gap in nutrition education and recognize the value of cooking to optimizing epigenetic inputs of diet. Dr. Shad founded the Culinary Medicine Program at the University of Arizona Medical with the goal of expanding education in nutrition by exposing students to both the art of cooking and the science of food as medicine. Culinary medicine involves teaming up with local chefs and farmers to connect patients and physicians with food, and teaches them how to prepare meals that optimize our health. Culinary medicine empowers both doctors and their patients to unlock the potential of food as an epigenetic input. With meal planning and innovative recipes, doctors can target medical conditions, optimizing health regimens to prevent disease and boost immunity and wellness.

By introducing programs like this into medical education, we can fill the gap of nutrition knowledge that most physicians have despite the key role that diet plays in our health and well-being. By training future physicians and health professionals, patients and communities are empowered to utilize food as medicine to prevent and treat the diseases of our time. Students are educated on the impact of food

---

policy on health, and how they can work as advocates in their communities to change our food system and thus improve health outcomes for all. In order to grow this transformative program, the goal is to bring together chefs, farmers, policymakers, and health professionals to redesign medical education to create a science-based, four-year nutrition curriculum that includes community-based projects to address the social determinants of health. To learn more about the national impact of culinary medicine, visit the Teaching Kitchen Collaborative, an organization that is working to catalyze and empower a growing network of innovators changing lives through food.

The Science of Nutrition: Your Diet Can Heal You—or Kill You

Many people believe they can simply take a medication to address some disease or ailment, but doing so without changing a poor diet is ultimately both ineffective and dangerous. For example, I remember one of my patients, Ann, who had acid reflux and started taking Prilosec. Prilosec is part of a class of medications known as a proton pump inhibitor (PPI). Ann stayed on the PPI for years without making any lifestyle changes. PPIs are notorious for increasing our risk for osteoporosis, pneumonia, as well as deficiencies in vitamin B12 and magnesium. Ann, unfortunately, was hospitalized with pneumonia, which nearly killed her, before I met her. She also had osteopenia, the beginning of osteoporosis. I worked with Ann to stop her PPI and make healthy lifestyle changes to prevent her reflux symptoms with an occasional Tums, which also improved her calcium intake. With these changes, along with optimizing her dietary intake of calcium, supplementing with vitamin D, and doing weight-bearing activities, not only did Ann not develop osteoporosis, but she reversed her osteopenia.

Years of research, hundreds of thousands of studies, and a growing understanding of epigenetics are teaching us that food can be used therapeutically to treat and even help reverse many diseases. Heart disease, diabetes, cancer, and noninfectious chronic obstructive lung disease account for seven out of every ten deaths and more than 75 percent of all healthcare costs.[8] So, what role does diet play in these chronic conditions?

How Diet Affects Heart Disease

Let's start with heart disease, which includes high blood pressure, high cholesterol levels, and metabolic syndrome (a cluster of conditions, including high blood pressure, high blood sugar, excess body fat at the waistline, and abnormal cholesterol levels—and a key risk factor for both diabetes and heart disease). One study found that a whopping 45.4 percent of all metabolic and heart-related deaths could be prevented by addressing nutritional risk factors, such as excess sodium (salt) and a lack of nuts, seeds, and healthy fats in one's diet.[9] We've seen this result firsthand as well. I have seen patients lower their blood pressure and treat their cholesterol without medication by simply changing their diet and being more physically active. Extensive research has shown how a whole, plant-based diet high in fiber and rich in antioxidants can literally reverse plaque formation in the coronary arteries that supply blood to our heart. Healthy fats like those found in nuts, seeds, and extra-virgin olive oil have also been shown to treat and prevent heart disease.

How Diet Affects Cancers

According to the World Health Organization, as many as one-third of all cancers and more than 70 percent of certain cancers (such as colon cancer) can be prevented by proper diet and nutrition. A recent large prospective study (which tracks its participants over a long period of time) showed that a 10 percent increase in the proportion of ultra-processed food in diet was associated with an 11 percent increase in overall cancer risk and a 10 percent increase in breast cancer, specifically.[10] Ultra-processed foods are foods made in factories. I call these food-like substances *Frankenfoods* and will describe them in more detail later in this chapter.

Another study looked at men with prostate cancer. It was discovered that plant-based diets and lifestyle changes, including exercise, meditation, and group sessions for social support, altered gene expression within a matter of three months. After three months, 48 genes crucial to suppressing cancer growth were more active, while 453 genes that have been shown to promote cancer growth were found to be less active. Along with these gene changes, prostate cancer activity and tumor size decreased as well.[11]

How Diet Affects Diabetes

Type 2 diabetes, caused by insulin resistance, accounts for more than 95 percent of all diabetes. The link between type 2 diabetes and diet is inextricable. Diet is a major causal factor and a critical therapy for preventing, treating, and even reversing this devastating disease.

As seen with Miguel and his family, diabetes is not a death sen-[12]tence and can be reversed. I had the privilege of successfully treating many patients with type 2 diabetes with food as medicine. I remember another patient—we'll call him Bob—who came to see me when he was forty-five years old and weighed more than three hundred pounds. He had type 2 diabetes. His triglyceride level (which measures a type of fat in the bloodstream) was 1,600 (normal is below 150). His average blood sugar level was 400 (normal is about 100). And his A1C (which measures average blood sugar levels) was 11 (normal is less than 5.7). So he was off all the charts, and many doctors would have simply put him on insulin.

I didn't want to do that since Bob was committed to changing his eating habits, which, at the time, consisted of either fast food or sumptuous business dinners of very rich foods and drinks. I did prescribe medications to lower his high cholesterol and triglycerides, but then we talked about his diet. Bob didn't realize what foods were contributing to these high levels, so we reviewed everything he was eating. Over the next three months, he changed his diet and lost fifteen pounds, his triglycerides came down to 260, and his A1C decreased from 11 to 6. By six months, he had lost another twenty-five pounds, and after a year, he had lost sixty pounds. We had reversed his type 2 diabetes.

How Diet Influences Premature Preventable Deaths

In the United States, according to several long-term analyses from 1990 to 2016, dietary factors have been identified as the top risk factors for both *disability-adjusted life years* (which simply means the number of years that are lost because of ill health, disability, or early death) and *premature preventable death* (which are early deaths that could have been prevented by lifestyle changes, including losing weight and not smoking, which are the most common risk factors).[13] Globally, an analysis of the health effects of dietary risk factors from 1990 to 2017 in 195 countries found suboptimal diet to be responsible for more deaths than any other risks, including tobacco smoking, thus highlighting the urgent need to address diet around the world. Based on all these findings, nutrition is obviously a critical component of what determines your health.[14]

With this new scientific evidence, you can think of food as a messenger of information that signals literally thousands of your genes to turn on or off within a matter of weeks, depending on your dietary choices. Every time you eat, you provide information as epigenetic inputs that change the expression of your genes. During the fifteen to twenty days it takes your taste buds to turn over, you can literally shift the expression of thousands of genes and update your epigenetic software in a way that profoundly impacts your health.[15] At the end of this chapter, I will show you how you can test this with your own diet.

What You Eat Matters: The Difference Between Real Food and Frankenfoods

To optimize your system to prevent disease and stay healthy, you need to optimize your epigenetic inputs. Nutrition is a key epigenetic input. What you eat matters, so let's turn to the question of what to eat. What messages with different types of information do different kinds of food send to your genes? What are you eating now? To understand this better, let's start with the concept of *real food*.

Real food is something that has not been manufactured in a factory. It usually comes out of the ground and sometimes can include animals that eat things that come out of the ground. That may sound glib, so here are a few examples:

- *Real food includes all fruits*: apples, apricots, bananas, blackberries, blueberries, cantaloupe, cherries, clementines, cranberries, dates, dragon fruits, figs, grapes, grapefruits, guavas, honeydew, kiwis, kumquats, lemons, limes, lychees, mandarins, mangoes, nectarines, oranges, papayas, peaches, pears, persimmons, pineapples, plums, pomegranates, raspberries, star fruits, strawberries, tangerines, and watermelon—and any other fruit you can find or grow!

- *Real food includes all vegetables*: artichokes, asparagus, avocados, beets, bok choy, broccoli, Brussels sprouts, cabbage, carrots, cauliflower, celery, collard greens, corn, cucumbers, eggplants, garlic, green beans, kale, leeks, lettuce, lima beans, mushrooms, okra, onions, parsnips, peas, peppers, potatoes, radishes, rhubarb, romaine, rutabagas, scallions, spinach, squash, sweet potatoes, tomatoes, turnips, water chestnuts, yams, and zucchini—and any other vegetable you can grow or buy!

- *Real food includes all nuts*: almonds, Brazil nuts, cashews, filberts, hazelnuts, macadamia nuts, peanuts (which are actually legumes but are classified as nuts because of their similarity to other nuts), pecans, pine nuts, pistachios, walnuts, and many more.

- *Real food includes all seeds*: chia seeds, flax seeds, poppy seeds, pumpkin seeds, sesame seeds, sunflower seeds, to name just a few.

- *Real food includes wild seafood*: salmon, mackerel, herring, sardines, and anchovies, to name a few healthier seafood options.

- *Real food includes a few animals that eat things that come out of the ground*: To be clear, none of us need meat to be healthy, especially if we choose to eat a whole-food, plant-based or plant-forward (> 85 percent plant-based) diet, plus wild seafood. However, if you do choose to eat meat, less is more, and the quality is even more important. For example, even in the Blue Zones, the diets are predominantly plant-based, and meat is limited to the size of a deck of cards up to four or five times per month. And the meat you should eat should be real—in other words, if you eat red meat that comes from cows or lamb, these should be pasture-raised and grass-fed without processing and the addition of chemicals and large quantities of antibiotics.

If all of the above are "real foods," then what is *not* real?

Fake foods, which I like to call Frankenfoods that masquerade as food, are not real foods. These food-like substances are mostly manufactured in a factory and contain additives, chemicals, and other processing elements to form a product. These products may have elements of real food, such as parts of a potato or meat, but they are loaded with other ingredients that are not actually food. Most prepackaged foods and processed foods are Frankenfoods. Almost all fast foods are also Frankenfoods because of the long list of chemical ingredients and processing methods used to produce them.

I'm not being harsh when I categorize these food-like substances as Frankenfoods; instead, they're in this category because the other chemical ingredients in them do not provide any nutritional benefit—and, in fact, in most cases, they are harmful to your health. These Frankenfoods also come loaded with excess amounts of refined sugar and excess sodium that disrupt our immune systems and contribute to chronic inflammation. While these food-like substances are high in calories, they are also woefully low in healing nutrients. This distorted version of real food is the root cause of the diseases of our time.

For example, candy bars and packaged treats are Frankenfoods that have been manipulated and distorted, resulting in negative health outcomes. Hydrogenated oils are a common ingredient in many of these (and other) processed foods. These oils increase the shelf life of these products, so they can be sold to customers (that means *you*) for six months or longer after they are produced. Although this makes financial sense to companies in the food industry, it is not so good for you from a health perspective.

Here's the science behind the use of hydrogenated oils: They are created by using high temperatures and pressures to force a hydrogen atom on the carbon backbone of an oil to stabilize that fat. This damages the fat, and damaged fat contributes to oxidation or damage of LDL cholesterol. LDL damage triggers an inflammatory response—and this inflammation is the first step in the process of atherosclerosis or narrowing of the arteries. Years of eating processed foods with hydrogenated oils will repeatedly oxidize and damage your LDL, leading eventually, because of narrowed arteries, to a heart attack or stroke.

The Standard American Diet Is SAD

Figure 4.2 shows a simple breakdown of the Standard American Diet (SAD), which is, quite frankly, *sad:* You can see that ultra-processed Frankenfoods account for up to (or even more than) 60 percent of all calories consumed.[16] As the data accumulates, we are learning more about how the food industry is like the tobacco industry in creating addictive products that manipulate your taste buds and contribute to the chronic diseases of our time. There is now consensus that poor diet is a larger contributor to the burden of noncommunicable chronic disease than tobacco, alcohol, and inactivity combined.[17]

The Standard American Diet

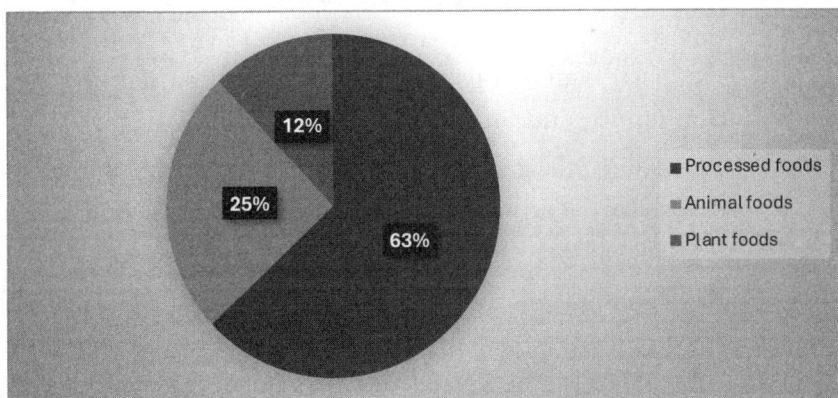

Adapted from U.S. Department of Agriculture, Agricultural Research Service and the U.S. Department of Health and Human Services, Centers for Disease Control and Prevention. What We Eat in America, NHANES 2001-2004 or 2005-2006.

One of the things we're learning about Frankenfoods is how they trigger inflammation in your body at a molecular level. Chemically, *cytokines* are released (as messenger molecules sending a kind of "SOS") in response to the perceived "damage" that these processed foods bring with them, leading to a low-grade inflammatory response. This is exactly the kind of toxic, chronic inflammation I discussed in Chapter 3. As I said earlier, although short-term inflammation (as seen with cuts and bruises) is a key part of the healing response, long-term inflammation directly contributes to the development of chronic disease.

What's Wrong with the SAD Standard American Diet

- **High in bad fats:**
  - Processed industrialized seed oils—such as soybean, corn, or canola oil
  - Trans fats—which are found in almost all commercially baked cakes, processed forms of bread, cookies, and pies; microwave popcorn; frozen pizza; refrigerated dough for biscuits and rolls; fried foods such as fried chicken, doughnuts, and French fries; and stick margarine.
  - Partially hydrogenated fats—which are found in potato chips, corn chips, nondairy coffee creamers, and other foods.

- **High in omega-6 fatty acids**: Intake of omega-6 fatty acids has doubled in the last one hundred years due to increased use of corn oil, safflower oil, and refined soybean oil in processed foods.

- **High in high-glycemic-load carbohydrates**: Foods made with lots of flour, sugar, and high-fructose corn syrup lead to chronic inflammation and promote insulin resistance in many people (which leads to diabetes). For example, sugar and sugary foods, such as commercially baked cookies, cakes, and pies; sugary soft drinks (sodas); and white bread.

- **High in additives**: Artificial food colorings and altered ingredients (such as aspartame, the artificial sweetener sold under brand names like NutraSweet® and Equal®), which are associated with a variety of mental and physical illnesses.

- **Low in good fats**: Intake of omega-3 fatty acids, especially anti-inflammatory, anti-thrombotic omega-3 fatty acids primarily found in extra-virgin olive oil, avocados, nuts, seeds, as well as in oily, wild, cold-water fish (such as salmon, mackerel, or sardines), has decreased to less than 20 percent of what was present in common diets 150 years ago.

- **Low in plant foods**: Fruits and vegetables are the main dietary sources of protective antioxidants and plant-based nutrients; most of us get very little of these that make up only about 12 percent of the SAD.

- **Low in protective micronutrients**: Vitamin D and magnesium[18], found in nuts, seeds, mushrooms, and cold-water fish, are lacking in many American diets.

Real food as opposed to Frankenfood is not mass-produced for short-term commercial gain, as is the case with what most Americans eat.

Americans' typical diet is low in what you should be eating more of and high in what you should be eating less of. The SAD is woefully low in whole vegetables and whole fruits which are the main source of fiber that feeds our microbiome to keep us healthy. Dominated by processed foods, the SAD is excessively high in unhealthy fats (processed seed oils and hydrogenated oils and fake butters like margarine) and sugars, refined grains (such as white breads, crackers, and pastries), and sodium, and it is slightly higher than ideal for saturated fat (which is found, for example, in fatty cuts of meat, sausages, bacon, salami and other processed meats and cheeses). This high-calorie, nutrient-poor diet is literally a recipe for metabolic disaster.

Our diet in the United States is low in whole, plant-based foods like dark green vegetables, beans, legumes, and vegetables. While it is low in whole grains that are loaded with fiber, it is much higher than recommended in refined grains that are simple sources of sugar, contributing to diabetes and obesity.

When you consider eating processed foods, you must understand that these foods have been manufactured deliberately to manipulate your taste buds and hijack your hormones to form addictions to them. It has been argued that sugar, especially in the excess amounts found in most processed foods, can be addictive. There is a commercial advantage for the food industry in making products such as soda and candy bars addictive. Most of these processed foods are high in sugar without fiber (discussed in detail in the carbohydrate section of this chapter), which has a range of negative epigenetic implications for your body.

Excess salt is also something that your taste buds crave, so most of these Frankenfoods are high in sodium as well. In fact, processed food is filled with tons of flavors that are developed in laboratories to create cravings. In nature, most flavors are associated with certain nutrients. When animals in the wild crave sweet or salty flavors, they are doing so because their system gets the flavorless nutrient that is in the plants or foods they eat. For example, lycopene (a plant-based nutrient with health benefits) in tomatoes is flavorless, but tomatoes have a certain flavor, so people who love the taste of tomatoes enjoy what they're eating and get the health benefits of lycopene at the same time, even though that has nothing to do with their craving for the tomato's flavor.

By separating flavor from nutrients, processed Frankenfoods have created a low-nutrient, high-flavor food industry. As you are exposed to more flavors, you crave them. Sadly, no nutrients come with these flavors. For instance, the chips that are bean- and salsa-flavored don't have the fiber or plant-based nutrients that are actually found in real beans and tomatoes. So you keep eating instinctually, without getting the nutrients your body is craving. This creates a bottomless pit, where you continually eat these "empty" calories devoid of nutrients to fill a hole that can never be filled. Epigenetics is working against you when these food-like substances fool your body into wanting more and more of them. Your good genes turn off and your bad genes turn on, leading to obesity, diabetes, and all the diet-related diseases of our time.

Why do most of us eat in this SAD way? Why are such unhealthy processed foods with these excess sugars and bad fats such a large part of the SAD in the United States? Why are organically produced fruits and vegetables relatively more expensive than fast foods?

One main reason for all of this is the broken food system in the United States. Ever wonder why fast food, which is the ulti-mate processed Frankenfood, is so cheap and widely available, while vegetables and plant-based healthy foods are so much more expensive? Are vegetables simply rarer and harder to find? Do they intrinsically take more resources to grow than to manufacture, for example, two-liter bottles of soda? They are hard to find on the plates of most Americans!

But the reason they don't make it to the plate has less to do with a desire for folks to eat healthy, and more to do with the barriers to healthy eating. These barriers inadvertently started back in 1933 with the passage of the original Farm Bill to provide federal sub-sidies for certain crops over others. Appendix A provides a more complete discussion of this topic, which is beyond the scope of the basics you need to know now about diet.

Recognizing that the food system is broken is an important part of understanding how to fix it. On a community level, part of the solution is to support local agriculture and innovative initiatives advocating for reform of the system. Individually, changing your diet to optimize epigenetic inputs from food not only has many health benefits, it can also contribute to a better food system by vot-ing with your fork, one bite at a time. Let's take a closer look at two types of food: red meat and plants.

Red Meat: Mass-Produced versus Grass-Fed

One example of a Frankenfood is highly processed, mass-produced meat versus traditionally pasture-raised, grass-fed meat. I believe you do not need to eat any meat to be healthy, and as I said before, less is more when it comes to meat; however, if you are going to eat meat, at least know the difference between real meat and processed Frankenfood versions of meat.

Real meat comes from animals that are treated well and given the diet they were evolved to eat for thousands of years. For example, cows have multiple stomachs to digest grass, which is their primary food. When you feed cows grain (instead of or in addition to grass), they become bigger and fatter more quickly, which is advantageous from a short-term economic perspective; in other words, the farmer makes more money from those cows.

However, feeding cows grain is not beneficial for the cow's health—or for human health. Grain-based diets in cattle are lower in healthy fats and antioxidants, and they have a much higher proportion of E. coli infections that can impact humans. (These are the stories we read in the news from time to time about a beef recall by a meat-packing plant, grocery store, or restaurant whose customers have experienced severe stomach cramps, diarrhea, or vomiting— sometimes even resulting in death, especially in young children.) Grain-fed meat is also higher in LDL cholesterol and lower in omega-3 fatty acids (an essential anti-inflammatory fat for brain and heart health).

Furthermore, grass-fed meat is better for the environment, according to several ecological indicators. The opposite is true for meat from grain-fed cows. In addition to using grain feed, mass meat production also uses other animals as part of the feed. That's right! Cows are being forced to engage in cannibalism by eating other cows and parts from other animals as a standard part of meat manufacturing in the United States. (That's what led to mad cow disease, which is fatal in cows and in humans who eat meat from cows with this disease.)

Now, no doctor will recommend that you eat red meat daily—not even "real" red meat. It is not the best source of calories in your diet, and it increases your risk for colon cancer, heart disease, and inflammation, leading to other debilitating conditions. However, if you are going to consume it, less is more, and eating the "real" form, which is from grass-fed cows, is a healthier option. This is an example of a real food versus a Frankenfood, which is a big part of the diet that most Americans consume every day.

Plants: Genetically Modified Organisms (GMOs) versus Organic

Another factor in recognizing a Frankenfood is the presence of GMOs. Plants have been bred, crossbred, and, therefore, "genetically" modified, for literally thousands of years. Crossing certain strains resulted in bigger fruits, sweeter fruits, or whatever we desired, depending on human interest. (For example, the maize that was grown thousands of years ago was higher in protein, higher in fiber, and lower in carbohydrates, whereas the corn we eat today has been selected and modified and is now much higher in carbs, lower in fiber, and lower in protein—which is why we use it for corn syrup.)

The difference with modern-day genetic modification is that we add non-plant elements to plants. An example of this is adding genes that code to produce pesticides in plants to protect them from invading insects. While this may sound like a good idea, we have no idea what impact this modification can have. Ecologically, how will this impact the careful balance of pathogens and plants in the environment? Will the plant still draw nutrients adequately from the soil to protect itself by building up its immunity to pathogens—or will the plant now become less nutrient-dense as a result of this modification? What are the potential dangers of excess pesticide concentration in conventionally produced produce?

Studies have shown that organic, non-GMO plants have lower levels of pesticides than conventionally produced fruits and vegetables. Some studies have even shown nonorganic produce to be lower in nutrients than organic produce. There is also the question of how these genetic modifications impact human gut health or the microbiome.

The main point about GMOs is this: Some may be fine, but others could be harmful, and researchers have not adequately considered all the potential implications from an evolutionary biology perspective to know for sure. Yet, despite this, GMOs have been added to your food supply mostly because of the drive to produce quick-yield, high-profit returns without a complete analysis of the long-term consequences. As organics can be more expensive, I recommend using evidence-based guides to decide which organic products to buy based on the potential for pesticide concentration.

For example, the Environmental Working Group's (EWG) recommendations on what organic fruits and vegetables to buy is based on its independent research on pesticide concentrations in these plants. The EWG has created something called the "Dirty Dozen," which are the twelve plant foods (such as berries and leafy greens) that have the highest concentration of pesticides and therefore are best to buy organic. Alternatively, the EWG has also compiled the "Clean 15," which are fifteen produce items that are conventionally grown containing the least amount of pesticides. For more information, you can visit its website at https://www.ewg.org/ for the latest information and guidelines.

Macronutrients: What You Need to Know about Carbs, Fats, and Proteins

Now that I have discussed the difference between real food and Frankenfood and the broken food system that has set us up for failure, let's look at macronutrients. These are the major types of calories in your diet—namely carbohydrates, fats, and proteins. Let's break down each of the excessive elements in our highly processed food diet as a way to understand where macronutrients fit in to your diet and dispel some of the most popular myths involved.

Are Carbs Good or Bad?

Carbohydrates are simple or complex starches or sugars. Naturally occurring sources of carbs include starchy vegetables (potatoes, sweet potatoes, corn, beets, squash, turnips, and others), and most fruits. Almost all Frankenfoods (even those you may not expect, such as baked beans) have high levels of refined carbohydrates in them. Most of this is in the form of added sugars and refined grains, like those found in white bread and pastries.

One of the main contributors to the diet-related diseases of our times is the high amount of refined sugar or simple carbs in the SAD. Also, if you look around the world where SAD and other Western diets have replaced traditional cultural diets, the additional refined sugar and refined grains in Western diets results in increased rates of obesity, diabetes, and heart disease, all contributing to premature disease and death in those countries as well as in the United States. For instance, type 2 diabetes, which is caused by excess simple sugars or refined carbs in the diet without fiber, is the leading cause of non-congenital blindness, kidney failure, and lower limb amputation; these outcomes are what we can prevent in people like Miguel who are able to use food as medicine to reverse their diabetes.

Because of what we now know about excess refined carbohydrates in our diet, many people argue that all carbs are bad. Some famous biohackers have written extensively about this, and it is also part of some popular diets, including the ketogenic diet. So, is it fair to demonize all carbohydrates as a bad thing?

The answer, based on what we know, is both yes and no. Yes, we eat way too much sugar in the form of refined grains and simple carbs in our highly processed food diets. And yet, no, not all forms of carbs are bad for you.

Let's break this down a bit more. Carbs can be simple and refined, or complex and unrefined. Here are some examples:

- brown rice (complex) versus white rice (simple)
- whole grain (unrefined) bread versus white or wheat (refined) bread
- whole fruits versus fruit juice

In short, you should eat more of the complex, unrefined, whole plant foods in the above list, and less (or none) of the simple or refined foods in the list. The key difference here is fiber. Real foods that are higher in complex carbohydrates or complex sugars (such as fruits) also tend to be higher in fiber. For example, dates are very high in sugar, but they are also extremely fibrous. That's why some studies have shown that eating a moderate amount of whole dates not only does not increase our risk for diabetes; it can actually help lower our blood sugar, and total cholesterol and triglyceride levels. Oranges are another example. So, let's dispel this myth about carbs being all bad. Orange juice in excess can be bad, but eating whole oranges is usually good.

Let's take the example of squeezing a glass of orange juice. Try this at home! How many oranges does it usually take for you to squeeze enough to fill an entire glass with juice? The answer is at least five or six, depending on the size of the glass and how juicy your oranges are. Now, take those same oranges and peel and eat them whole. Remember, you must chew up all the fibrous tissue parts of the fruit (you can't spit it out!). Now, how many oranges can you eat before you start to feel full? The answer likely drops to one to two oranges. The reason is the fiber in the whole fruit versus the juice.

In nature, any plant-based food that is sweet, like fruit, is also high in fiber. When you eat whole fruits, the fiber expands in your stomach, resulting in a mechanical stretch of your stomach, sending a signal back to the brain that you are feeling "full." In addition to this mechanical change to control your portion size by signaling satiety or fullness, it also takes longer for the sugar to be digested when it's attached to fiber, resulting in a slower rise in blood sugar levels as opposed to the big jump in levels after you drink juice. That big bump in blood sugar from juice leads to a bump in insulin, which leads to more sugar being changed into fat.

Over time, repeated bursts of high-sugar, low-fiber foods (basically most processed foods and sugary beverages) can lead to insulin resistance, which in turn leads to diabetes, increased fat production, and obesity. The excess weight and higher uric-acid levels with higher insulin levels also lead to higher blood pressure. And the excess sugar that isn't used up with physical activity turns into bad fat, specifically triglycerides. All of these increase your risk of heart disease, heart attacks, and strokes. New evidence also shows a relationship between chronically elevated insulin levels, chronic inflammation, and cancer risk.

There is also evidence of the long-term health benefits of having a diet that is higher in complex carbohydrates. Plant-based diets—such as vegan and vegetarian diets—are both much higher as a percentage of total calories in carbohydrates as compared to ketogenic or low-carb diets. Both vegan and vegetarian diets are associated with lower rates of diet-related diseases across the board, including obesity, heart disease, diabetes, cancer, markers of chronic inflammation, premature aging, and premature death.

The key here is that vegetarians and vegans who eat real food also avoid processed foods, which are high in refined carbs. Most carbohydrates eaten by vegetarians and vegans are complex carbohydrates that are not refined, such as whole-grain bread, whole vegetables, and brown rice. These complex carbohydrates are loaded with fiber—in fact, plant-based diets are the highest in fiber content. This leads to all the protective benefits that fiber provides, including lowering the risk for heart disease, colon cancer, diabetes, and obesity, and improving overall gut health.

Fiber can lower bad cholesterol levels, lower blood pressure, improve our digestion, prevent and help treat diabetes, and even help prevent colon cancer. Furthermore, fiber is also the main food for the microbiome, which is composed of all the good bacteria in our gut, nasal passages, mouth, and lungs. These good bacteria outnumber human cells. In fact, we are 90 percent bacteria and only 10 percent human.

Emerging research has shown that the health of the microbiome is a critical piece of the diseases of our time. Microbiome diversity protects you from disease. Researchers have traveled to undeveloped parts of the world where people eat more traditional, higher-fiber diets to study those people's microbiomes. They took stool samples and found much more diversity compared to samples from people in more developed countries.

One reason for this is how little fiber Americans typically eat. Unfortunately, the SAD is low in fiber, the main food of the microbiome. This has led to a narrowing of diversity in microbiome species that has been associated with obesity, diabetes, heart disease, premature aging, and several forms of cancer.

Do extremely low-carb diets work? And if so, how? We all know people who have successfully lost weight by cutting out the carbs. The main reason this works in the United States is that you are eliminating excess carbs in the form of sugar, which is a huge part of the SAD. This is not only true in the United States, but also in any part of the world where similar diets have been adopted to replace healthier traditional diets. For example, the ketogenic diet, in its pure form, has most calories consumed from fat, not protein, and very low amounts from carbs. You can see how shifting epigenetic input from a high-refined-carb diet to a very low-carb diet can have dramatic changes in terms of weight, blood pressure, and other health parameters.

Debunking Myths about Fats

Another macronutrient is fat. For many decades, fats were demonized as the main cause of heart disease and intuitively thought to make people fat. This led to a whole generation of people avoiding all fat as much as possible. The food industry followed suit with this dogma and created a whole range of fat-free and low-fat products. The American Heart Association became convinced of the crimes of fat based on what health professionals now recognize as misunderstood research from Ancel Keys, a physiologist who argued that saturated fat caused heart disease.

Here, we have another case similar to our discussion about carbohydrates, where the truth is more complex. It is similarly complicated with fats as with carbs—that is, not all fats are bad. In fact, you need certain good fats for both brain and heart health.

To simplify this, let's go back to the thirty-year mistake of advocating for a low-fat diet. Although there is data to support the negative impact of saturated fat on cardiovascular disease, there are two pitfalls that occurred with the low-fat diet. One has to do with what we ate instead of fat, and the other with fat itself.

First, the low-fat admonition led to the low-fat foods that replaced fat with various forms of sugar. Since we did not clearly recognize the role that refined carbohydrates played in the diet-related diseases of our time, those same three decades saw the greatest rise in diabetes and obesity because of the rise in sugar consumption. We learned from this that sugar is an epigenetic input that makes us fat. As noted above, excess refined sugar without fiber leads to chronically elevated levels of insulin. Insulin is the fat-forming and fat-storing hormone signaling our bodies to make more fat.

The second issue with the low-fat diet is that all fat is not actually bad. In fact, fat is critical to life. Most of your cells, including almost the entirety of your brain, are made up of fat. You need fat to survive. And certain kinds of fat—for example, monounsaturated fat—can contribute to weight loss. (You can find monounsaturated fat in avocados; nuts such as almonds, hazelnuts, and pecans; seeds such as pumpkin seeds and sesame seeds; and in extra-virgin olive oil or avocado oil.) Studies have shown diets higher in monounsaturated fats as a percentage of total caloric intake when controlling for total calories led to weight and fat loss.

One of the biggest head-to-head diet studies at the time between the standard American Heart Association low-fat diet and the Mediterranean Diet, high in fat, was stopped halfway through because the Mediterranean Diet group had huge health benefits, making it unethical to continue the study. This happens in clinical trials, when one intervention (in this case, the Mediterranean Diet) is found to be far superior to the other intervention (in this case, the standard [at the time] American Heart Association low-fat diet). The differences were so stunning that the entire medical community had to reevaluate what we thought we knew about fat. The main sources of healthy fat in the Mediterranean Diet that have been shown to have the most health benefits are monounsaturated fats from high-quality extra-virgin oil, tree nuts (pistachios, walnuts, almonds, pecans, and almonds), and wild seafood.

Subsequently, many research studies have now confirmed a more complicated picture of fat that endorses the benefits of the healthy fats found in the Mediterranean Diet for both primary and secondary prevention of heart disease. (Primary prevention is for people who don't have heart disease; although they may have a risk for it, they have not been diagnosed with it. Secondary prevention is for people who have had a heart attack or stroke or a diagnosis of heart disease, and they want to prevent further damage to the heart.)

In general, we have learned that there are both good and bad fats, as well as something in between. Plant-based fats (nuts, seeds, avocados, and olive oil) are by far the healthiest sources of fat. Other sources of healthy fat include wild fatty fish, such as salmon or mackerel. Saturated fat is both good and bad because it raises HDL ("good" cholesterol) and raises LDL ("bad" cholesterol). The monounsaturated fats and polyunsaturated fats (especially omega-3 fatty acids) all have a beneficial impact on cholesterol levels and health.

How Important Are Proteins?

Proteins are one of the main macronutrients in your body that contribute to your muscles, as well as to neurotransmitters in your nervous system. Protein is an essential building block of all cells; however, excess protein, especially from animal sources, can be harmful to the kidneys and promote weight gain. It is a myth that vegetarians and vegans cannot get adequate protein. There are plenty of excellent plant sources of protein, including, but not limited to, nuts, seeds, and legumes (such as beans, chickpeas, and lentils).

My friend and mentor, Dr. Christopher Gardner, nutrition professor at the Stanford School of Medicine, has written and spoken extensively about the myth of protein. In fact, the data shows that in the United States, we consume too much protein and too little fiber. There are more and more fully plant-based athletes, including body builders, who have high lean muscle mass from consuming all their protein from plant-based sources. Some research even suggests that close to 90 percent of muscle mass comes down to exercise, and only 10 percent is produced from getting adequate protein. Excess protein that is not broken down by exercise and used to rebuild muscle cannot be stored; it is converted to sugar or fat. So it is a good idea to continue resistance and weight training exercise (more on this in the Exercise chapter) to maintain muscle mass and slow down aging over time.

Biochemically, what distinguishes protein from other macronutrients is nitrogen. Some proteins and amino acids cross the blood-brain barrier and can influence our moods. The blood-brain barrier is a protective natural barrier between your brain and the rest of your body. Certain chemicals in foods and drugs can cross this and affect your brain with anticipated and unintended consequences. For example, tryptophan is an essential amino acid, which means the body cannot make its own supply but must get it from food. Tryptophan is a precursor for serotonin, which is a key neurotransmitter involved in your mood. Not having enough serotonin available can be the main chemical cause of depression. That's why the most commonly prescribed antidepressant medications are selective serotonin reuptake inhibitors (SSRIs), which enhance your serotonin levels as a way of treating depression.

Proteins are important for muscle and structural needs in your body. Protein is also needed for healthy brain development, the ability for brains to adapt and create new neurons. Structural needs like skin, hair, and nails all require adequate protein levels in the diet. Protein is also a key part of any meal, in that it helps to signal that you are full, thereby controlling portion size and preventing you from eating too much. Protein is not an ideal source of energy, as it should be reserved for building blocks that are not broken down for fuel.

What You Should Know carbs, fats, and proteins.

Figure 4.5: What You Should Know about Carbs, Fats, and Proteins

Macro-nutrient	Myths Debunked	The Best	The Worst	Key Points
Carbohy-drates	Not all carbs are bad; excess simple/refined carbs can make us sick, while fiber-rich complex carb sources keep us healthy.	Naturally occurring with fiber in whole grains and non-starchy vegetables/leafy greens; best in complex unrefined state.	Excess refined carbs and simple carbs lead to diet-related diseases like diabetes, obesity, and heart disease, and increase risk for certain cancers.	Stick to unrefined complex carbs; SAD is high in refined carbs, so avoid Frankenfoods and limit simple or refined carbs.
Fats	Fat is essential for health. The key is good fat versus bad fat; we need good fat for brain and heart health.	Best are undamaged, unprocessed healthy fats that are found in plant foods (nuts, seeds, avocado, extra-virgin olive oil), and wild seafood.	Worse are hydrogenated oils, trans fat, and processed fats that are damaged, like industrially produced seed oils; saturated fat can be good and bad.	Eat healthy fats and avoid bad fats. Monounsaturated fats are the best fats, followed by omega-3 fatty acids, found in walnuts, flaxseed or fish oil (wild cold-water fish).

| Proteins | Vegetarians and vegans DO get enough protein. You do not need animal protein to thrive. | Best protein comes from plant sources (e.g. peas, beans, and lentils). If animals are eaten, less is more; choose grass-fed / pasture-raised meats. | Minimal to no animal sources. Avoid processed meat and mass-produced meat, as these can be cancer causing and contribute to heart disease. | Avoid excess protein; choose primarily plants and seafood sources; if you eat animal sources, make sure they are all unprocessed. |

How Much of Each Macronutrient Should I Eat?

This all depends on the type of diet you eat and the form of the macronutrient. For example, a whole-food, plant-based diet like the vegan diet will inevitably be much higher in carbohydrates. However, the source of carbohydrates is always whole plants, such as whole vegetables and fruits, which are sources of abundant antioxidants that reduce inflammation and fiber that balances blood sugar and feeds our microbiome. If you eat a ketogenic diet, a whopping 70 percent of your calories need to come from fat, followed by 20 percent from protein, and 10 percent from carbohydrates. This diet, like any diet that is not the Standard American Diet, has been shown to have benefits for weight, blood pressure, and cholesterol. However, the source and quality of the fat is important. Getting this from mostly plant sources like avocado, nuts, seeds, and high-quality extra-virgin olive oil (EVOO) is better than processed meats and unhealthy processed fats.

Another key point here is how the combination of macronutrients can help optimize health. For example, when looking to optimize blood sugar in people who are prediabetic or diabetic (together this accounts for more than 100 million people in the United States alone), combining healthy sources of carbs with healthy fats and proteins makes a huge difference. In many patients, like Miguel, I would advise a combination of healthy carb sources, such as a whole apple with a handful of tree nuts with healthy fat and protein. The whole apple versus the juice has fiber, which lowers blood sugar. When you combine this with a handful of nuts, the fat and protein further lower the glycemic load of the meal, resulting in lower blood sugar by slowing down the digestion of the food into simple sugars. Another example is whole-grain toast with avocado, EVOO, and nuts—or beans with avocado, nuts, and EVOO. The combination of quality sources for macronutrients can make a huge impact on a major disease like diabetes.

What You Can Do: Learn How to Read Nutrition Labels

One way to recognize processed food or Frankenfood versus real food is to read labels. The safest bet is to avoid prepacked foods altogether. I agree with the well-known author and journalist Michael Pollan, who calls these processed foods "edible food-like substances," and advises us to avoid prepackaged foods with more than five ingredients or with any ingredients you can't pronounce. This is a good general rule to follow when trying to verify that ingredients are real foods, rather than chemicals or added sugars that can wreak havoc on your system.

Since it isn't always practical to avoid eating prepackaged foods, you need to learn to read food labels.

Food labels can be confusing. Here are some helpful points to determine if this is something you should be eating:

- First, look at the ingredients list. As mentioned, if you don't recognize an ingredient as a real food, you shouldn't be eating it—or you should at least limit how much of this Frankenfood you eat.

- Next, look at the "Nutrition Facts" information, starting with the serving size. Serving sizes are often confusing, and you need to pay attention to see how much they are referring to: Is it the whole package, one-quarter of the package, or something else? This is important for understanding the referenced breakdown of macronutrients.

- When looking at the macronutrients, pay attention to a recent change in food labels that includes "Added Sugars." This allows consumers to see how much excess sugar has been added to the food. For example, a packaged food with fruits will have more carbohydrates and fiber that help to offset the sugar if it is not only juice. However, if there is added sugar listed, that means the food manufacturer added *more* sugar to what the fruit already had. This is something you want to avoid for many reasons, including the fact that most of us already get too much sugar, which is a big part of the processed Frankenfoods in our SAD.

Experiment with Your Own Diet: Eliminate Salt or Sugar for Three Weeks

Many of us have a sweet tooth or crave salty foods. But there is such a thing as too much of a tasty thing. In the Standard American Diet (SAD), we consume way too much salt and refined sugar in the processed foods we eat. Eliminating excess sodium in our diet is one of the main ways to prevent deaths from heart disease, obesity, diabetes, and even some forms of cancer. And excess sugar is a major contributor to obesity, diabetes, heart disease, and even some cancers.

There are two main reasons why sugar is so ubiquitous in our SAD. One is the Farm Bill, which makes sugar in all its processed forms so cheap and widely available that it's added to almost every processed food. The second reason is sugar's potential for addiction. The food industry has recognized this, and it is part of the reason why it is so useful in selling their Frankenfood products. Functional MRI studies have observed the areas of the brain that "light up" through stimulation from various substances. One study observed the impact of cocaine versus a lump of sugar; remarkably, the same areas of the brain lit up with both.[19] When you combine this human brain study with the numerous animal studies showing how addictive sugar is, you realize we have so much sugar in our SAD not by accident but by design to keep us buying these Frankenfood products. One of the first steps in using food as medicine in our society is to recognize sugar addictions and begin the process of getting people off sugar. The same can be said for the excess salt in our diets.

Thankfully, our taste buds change in just twenty-eight days. So, one DIY biohacking experiment you can do is to read labels, avoid Frankenfoods and all packaged foods for twenty-eight days. When it comes to salt, don't add salt during the cooking process; instead, limit your salt intake by only adding some salt to taste at the table. Also, try Himalayan pink salt or sea salt instead of standard table salt, because these types of salt are lower in sodium and also include some needed minerals, such as manganese. Look for added sugar on labels and avoid any products with added sugar and also any ingredients that include forms of sugar. Limit sugar to naturally occurring sugar in whole fruits and avoid fruit juices and sugary beverages.

After twenty-eight days, try eating something you ate before like a packaged food or a fast-food item that was part of your diet. You will find the taste of salt or sugar overwhelming, and you'll actually prefer the real foods you have been eating. Your taste buds have changed and adjusted to a new normal. You will also feel more energy and not have the usual crash that comes from the sugar high. You may even feel less bloated and lighter from the excess salt you were eating. Limiting excess sugar and salt will also lower your blood pressure and your blood sugar, help you lose weight, and experience fewer cravings for unhealthy Frankenfoods. Your immune system will also be boosted by avoiding excess sugar and salt, as both impair our immunity, leading to more frequent infections.

What's even more important is that your gene expression and software system has been updated and changed in a matter of weeks. When making a change, make sure to keep your diet for at least twenty-eight days to change your taste buds and your genes. This is epigenetics at work through biohacking using nutrition as an epigenetic input!

Final Thoughts on Diet

When considering any major dietary change, it's important to recognize that any change that incorporates more "real foods" would be better than the SAD that most Americans currently eat. When you embark on any dietary change, you will begin to consciously reflect on the food you eat. This shift is a big benefit, as it makes you think twice about what you put in your mouth. Some diet apps work well just by asking people to take pictures of their food. Sharing our diet makes us more self-conscious of what we eat.

As discussed, there are many reasons why it is easier for us to eat poorly. For many, it is because of cost, with food policy making unhealthy Frankenfoods cheap and widely available. For many, it is the addictive nature of these food-like substances, which have been manufactured by Big Food, to hook us for life on their unhealthy products. (Big Food refers to the major food manufacturing companies that, similar to Big Tobacco, produce food-like products that are addictive and unhealthy.) In this case, think of candy bars as sugar-delivery devices, just as cigarettes are nicotine-delivery devices, and you can see the parallel between Big Food and Big Tobacco.

For others, it is the path of least resistance because of being too "busy" to take the time to invest in buying and preparing healthy food. And fast food is just easier, now even more so with delivery apps that bring this food right to your door. Taking on a therapeutic diet often involves a more active role by actually planning, preparing, and even cooking your own meals. Cooking is a lost art for many people; in fact, fewer people cook at home now than they did forty years ago.[20] But cooking from basic real-food ingredients is a key investment in ensuring a diet that enhances your health and longevity. This is how culinary medicine works, where families and communities come together to cook meals that are delicious and nutritious. And studies now suggest that cooking more at home could have a number of health benefits.

There is much more to discuss regarding diet in the DRESS Code; I couldn't include all of it in this chapter. Therefore, in the chapters ahead, I will continue to consider diet as part of the whole picture that leads to reprogramming your genes for a healthier, longer life.

Key Points about Diet

> Food is a critical epigenetic input that can upgrade your genetic software to health or downgrade it to disease.

> Recognize the difference between real food and food-like substances, also known as Frankenfoods, that masquerade as food.

> By eating real food, you can begin to biohack and reprogram your genes to recognize how certain macronutrients work to heal us every day.

> Macronutrients—carbs, fat, and protein—are a key part of any diet. Their proportion, type, or source can be a critical input for health or disease.

> Carbohydrates can be both good and bad, depending on how much and what kind of carbohydrate you choose to eat. Carbs in processed foods are refined and in simple forms like sugar. These carbs lack fiber and can epigenetically drive bad software, resulting in obesity, heart disease, diabetes, and increased risk for many forms of cancer. Carbohydrates that are complex and unrefined are found in whole plant foods, which are fiber-rich and contribute to health.

> Fat can be good or bad. Good fat comes primarily from plant sources, including avocados, nuts, seeds, and certain oils,

such as extra-virgin olive oil. Plant-based fats can make you thin. Good fat also comes from wild, cold-water, fatty fish. Saturated fat can be both good and bad by raising our LDL and HDL cholesterol, making it a double-edged sword to eat in moderation as compared to monounsaturated fats (high in avocado, olive oil, pecans, and almonds) and polyunsaturated fats (especially the omega-3 fats found in walnuts, seaweed, and fatty fish).

➢ Protein is an essential building block of all cells, but excess protein, especially from animal sources, can be harmful to your kidneys and promote weight gain. Most of us eat too much protein, especially from animal sources. It is a myth that vegetarians and vegans cannot get adequate protein, because there are plenty of excellent plant sources of protein, including but not limited to nuts, seeds, and legumes.

➢ Not all calories are created equal. The source and type of calorie is important. Studies show that, even when controlling calorie count, changing the percentage of calories coming from different macronutrients can have a positive impact on your health.

➢ Genetically modified food is an experiment with some known dangers for consumers. Until more is known about these foods through unbiased independent research, it is best to avoid them as much as possible.

CHAPTER 5

R IS FOR RELATIONSHIPS: CONNECT TO THRIVE

The R in the DRESS Code is for relationships. Relationships— how we relate to others and the social world around us—are an epigenetic input just like diet and thus a key part of our health. When looking at relationships as epigenetic inputs, we find that the idea that we need one another to survive is even more important than we originally thought. As the well-known line from a poem by John Donne says, "No man is an island." The reality is that being socially isolated like an island without any meaningful relationships can negatively impact our health, just as connecting with others can help us not only to survive longer, but to thrive in all dimensions of life.

Human beings are social creatures. We require social interactions for many reasons. We learn basic skills of survival from our parents and the social cues around us as we develop in early life. Individuals who are impaired socially, such as from atypical neurological conditions like autism spectrum disorder (ASD), are limited in their ability to be successful in life. In such scenarios, we can see how a lack of social skills and the inability to connect can be disabling. Not being able to connect well with others is detrimental to everyone, not just those with disabling conditions.

Having emotional intelligence and connection with others allows us to enjoy and succeed at life. This can play out in different ways throughout our lives. In childhood, socialization is critical to healthy development, and the friendships we make allow us to grow in this meaningful part of life. As we enter adolescence and adulthood, finding others who share our values and perspective about the world is an important part of finding our place in the world. Such connections at every phase of life help make every task more enjoyable, leading to more engagement, learning, and growth for us. While connecting well with others can benefit our material success and even boost our mood, relationships are more important than that. The quality of our relationships can directly impact our physical health and longevity right down to the molecular level.

Relationships and Health

Relationships and the social aspects of life are a key epigenetic input, as evidenced by a large body of research that shows their impact on our well-being and health. Social support of some kind, be it in personal relationships or as part of a community, can prevent disease and enhance our ability to overcome it. Looking at relationships as an epigenetic input allows us to see how this unfolds at the molecular level. Everything we experience in life is an epigenetic input, upgrading our genetic software to achieve health or downgrading it to lead to disease and premature death.

A key part of the DRESS Code for Optimal Health includes relationships because our social connections are just as important as our diet, stress, and all the other epigenetic factors in influencing our health. Social inputs literally change our gene expression at the molecular level by upgrading or downgrading our software from within. This is the main reason why hundreds of studies have shown that people with more social ties live longer, healthier, and happier lives than those who are isolated without close ties to others. In fact, a review of more than 148 of these studies showed that people who lack social connections have 50 percent higher odds of dying than others who have strong social connections![21]

In one well-publicized Harvard study, people who were most satisfied with their relationships at age fifty were the healthiest at age eighty. This study, which followed more than seven hundred men since 1938, found that our satisfaction with our relationships at age fifty is a better predictor of our physical health than conventional objective measures like cholesterol levels. The Harvard study also found that these relationships were a better predictor of happiness than money or fame.[22] The significance of these findings is that happiness is not something we can achieve on our own, and neither is physical health. We have many individual choices we can make for healthy lifestyles, and being connected to others is one of those choices. The aging process, including the onset and progression of disease, can be potentially slowed down through the quality of our relationships.

Quality relationships do not necessarily need to be romantic. To connect meaningfully and authentically with others, we have to be willing to show vulnerability. Showing vulnerability—whether by sharing our weaknesses or challenges—is a key part of meaningful relationships. By showing this part of ourselves, we engender trust and build connections with others. Superficial friendships with so-called "fair weather" friends or relationships where vulnerability is not shared do not result in meaningful and authentic relationships.

Some of us are challenged by past traumas that create issues of trust that keep us from being vulnerable with others. It is important in these situations to process that trauma with the help of a mental health expert and use tools like eye movement desensitization and reprocessing (EMDR) or cognitive behavioral therapy (CBT). Working with an expert to learn how to show vulnerability and put yourself out there to create true friendships will have lasting impacts on your physical and mental health, as well as your ability to live healthier for longer.

One way to create meaningful, long-term relationships is marriage. Married people who have committed to a life partner have a higher life expectancy than unmarried people. Getting married can add three or more years to your life! There are many tangible and intangible benefits to being married. Some of the more intuitive benefits include having someone who can motivate us to stay healthy by engaging in healthy behavior. More intangible, or perhaps not always visible, is the molecular changes to our gene expression when we are not lonely that lead to enhanced immunity, reduced inflammation, and improved ability for us to be resilient through life's physical, emotional. and mental challenges.

A large body of literature now exists showing the benefit of support groups for a variety of medical conditions. This was first discovered among cancer survivors. Cancer patients who engage in regular support groups with other cancer survivors live longer and enjoy a higher quality of life. The very act of gathering with others who share our experiences can impact our health and well-being.

The concept of peer support has also been effective in managing and controlling chronic diseases like diabetes and heart disease. These programs involve peers connecting to share and learn from each other's successes and failures in living with a chronic medical condition. These groups have enabled patients to change their lifestyles to improve their quality of life, reduce objective risk factors like blood sugar levels, and reduce complications from diabetes.

You don't have to wait to have a chronic disease to connect with others for better health. You can start now by making time to connect meaningfully with others and create your own social groups. This could occur with any number of shared group activities, from a walking group to a regular game night—or even cooking together, as food connects us and can help us to build the community we need.

So, what makes relationships so beneficial? For one thing, relationships reduce stress levels by decreasing cortisol, a hormone related to stress. Reduction in stress translates into lowered blood pressure, improved immunity, and better regulation of insulin levels that can impact our risk for heart disease and diabetes. Imagine how simply hugging or cuddling with our dear ones can have a positive physiological impact on our health! For example, a hug lasting more than thirty seconds results in an almost instantaneous release of oxytocin, a hormone that can boost our moods, reduce the levels of harmful stress hormones in our bodies, and lower our blood pressure. When we further consider how cost effective it is to simply connect with others through touch in these simple ways, we can see how meaningful relationships should be encouraged for everyone as a key part of their healthcare strategy.

On the other hand, not having good relationships can be deadly. The impact of loneliness has recently been discovered to be a major contributor to our risk for disease and premature death. In fact, research has shown that the risk of loneliness is comparable to the risk of dying from smoking nearly fifteen cigarettes a day, and an even higher risk than being obese or physically inactive. Such research shows that loneliness, living alone with poor social connections, is worse than we previously understood. Being socially isolated without meaningful, regular social connections is deadly. Lonely people are more likely to suffer from several diseases, including mental health conditions like depression and medical conditions like heart disease and dementia.

In looking at the genes involved, research has shown that the same genes impacted by loneliness also code for immune function and inflammation. Therefore, loneliness can directly impact the downgrading of our software to weaken our immunity and increase inflammation. We've discussed how deadly chronic inflammation can be. The opposite is also thankfully true. Positive social experiences and connections create a positive feedback loop where we can experience mental, emotional, and physical well-being.

While there are times for us to be on our own and grow, social isolation is ultimately self-defeating. No matter how attentive you may be to all the other epigenetic inputs, such as diet and exercise, you can't cancel out the negative health impact of lacking meaningful relationships or social connections in your life. Some indicators suggest that loneliness itself can increase one's risk for death at any point by nearly 30 percent compared to people who are not lonely.

Unfortunately, loneliness or the lack of meaningful relationships is more common nowadays. Research from around the world has shown this to be worsening, especially after the onset of the COVID-19 pandemic. Globally, research has shown that 41 percent of people reported becoming lonelier during the course of the pandemic. Recent national survey data has shown that 36 percent of all Americans reported feeling lonely frequently or almost all the time—including 61 percent of young people ages eighteen to twenty-five and 51 percent of mothers with young children.[2324]

In this same survey, 43 percent of young adults reported worsening loneliness after the onset of the pandemic. Recently, even the Surgeon General of the United States released an advisory the American epidemic of loneliness and social isolation as a major public health concern. When considering the increased risks of disease and premature death associated with loneliness, as noted above, this staggering number represents a real epidemic of loneliness. Therefore, the presence or absence of relationships can upgrade or downgrade our software, leading to health or disease. Additionally, bad relationships can also serve as a negative epigenetic input on our health.

Social Media and Loneliness

Ironically, there is an epidemic of loneliness occurring in the era of social media. While it may seem that social media, by definition, should help us fill the void of social interactions to create positive relationships, it is actually now being recognized as a source of unhealthy relationships and even contributing to loneliness. In fact, much has been written about the toxicity of social media and how it is not a replacement for meaningful human interactions, be they in person or virtual.

Recent studies have shown that negative interactions on social media can lead to more feelings of social isolation and loneliness. Some studies have demonstrated a direct link between these negative interactions online and a clinically significant increased risk for depression. Contrary to what may seem like common sense, being active on social media does not count as having a positive relationship in your life. In fact, the highly scrutinized and critical environment of social media can provide a more toxic environment from unwelcomed interactions online.

These toxic interactions, at times with total strangers, are counterproductive and even lead to cyber forms of bullying and public shaming. People also tend to misrepresent themselves on social media, forming a near-perfect image of who they are that is far from the truth. This has led to a negative impact on mental health, and even suicide in some extreme cases.

Exercise caution when using social media. Make it a part of your day, but don't let it dominate your perceptions of yourself. And recognize the fact that social media can never replace meaningful authentic relationships in real life.

Toxic Relationships and Disease

Like other epigenetic inputs, good relationship inputs can lead to updated genetic software and better health. Bad relationship inputs can downgrade our software with malware, leading to poor gene expression and bad health.

In understanding relationships as an epigenetic input, we can see how good or bad relationships can have an impact on more than our psychological health. Toxic relationships, like toxic food, give us negative inputs that ultimately sabotage our system. This negative input creates the perfect setup for disease to occur. Toxic relationships are those that drag you down to where you are constantly in a state of conflict, disappointment, frustration, and sadness. While these negative states can occur in any relationship, the problem arises when they are persistent and without resolution despite professional intervention through counseling or therapy.

When this happens, it's time to recognize that the relationship may be a source of more harm than good in your life. Being in a toxic relationship, whether a romantic relationship or a professional one, has obvious implications for our mental health and our ability to enjoy our lives and be productive. However, recent research is now showing us that toxic relationships also have an impact on our physical health. Studies have demonstrated that being in a negative relationship can increase your risk for heart disease and having a fatal heart attack. One study of women with coronary artery disease found that increased marital stress was associated with a 2.9 percent increase in risk for a heart attack or stroke. Hostile relationships have even been shown to impact our immunity and our ability to heal from physical wounds!

Toxic relationships increase the baseline inflammation in our bodies. By increasing stress hormones and increasing resistance in our blood vessels, toxic relationships can literally kill us by contributing to the chronic inflammation that underlies the diseases of our time. These negative interactions can also inhibit our immune system, making us more susceptible to infections and certain cancers.

The Harvard study discussed earlier also found that those who were isolated and lonely or in unhappy marriages or relationships had an increased risk of memory problems, debilitating health, and premature death. Other studies have shown that the quality of our relationships matter. While many studies have shown that being married has a positive impact on our health, including a decreased risk for heart disease, some studies have also found unhappily married couples to experience negative health consequences. For example, one study found men who were unhappily married to be a whopping 86 percent more likely to die from sudden cardiac (heart-related) death as compared to men who were satisfied in their marriage.[25]

Our interactions with others can shape our gene expression and health. Research has also shown that negative interactions with friends or family are associated with poorer health. Again, the opposite is true as well. A large Swedish study looked at men and women ages sixty-five or older and found that those with the greatest satisfaction in their relationships with friends and relatives had the lowest risk of dementia. Poorer satisfaction, indicating unhealthy or toxic relationships, had the opposite effect.

Relationships in Communities

While meaningful individual relationships can be a powerful epigenetic input leading to health, many such connections form and develop in the context of communities. Communities of people who share the same values in the form of culture, social norms, or religion are another example of why relationships are a key part of the DRESS Code.

One key component for longevity and health in these settings is the absence of widespread loneliness and the presence of meaningful relationships stemming from a community of closely connected friends and family. The importance of these social bonds has been identified as a key element contributing to longevity and health in the Blue Zones.

One example is the Okinawan tradition of "Moais." Okinawans are among the longest-lived and healthiest communities in the world. Moais are groups of five friends who stay committed to each other throughout their entire lives. These groups are often formed deliberately by parents in the community during childhood. These groups provide social, financial, and spiritual support to one another through life. Like a support group, they meet regularly and form strong bonds. This part of their culture provides meaningful, authentic relationships as a part of life and is a major contributor to their longevity.

Staying connected with friends and investing in those relationships over time pays dividends down the road in terms of health and well-being. Studies show that smoking, obesity, happiness, and even loneliness are contagious, so the social networks of long-lived people have favorably shaped their health behaviors.

Being a part of a network of people who have shared values is one reason why communities are so important in cultivating healthy relationships. Whether your community is formed by a strong geographic neighborhood or by culture, the connections that come with belonging to any community are a natural place for good relationships to thrive. More than simply being an enjoyable part of one's life, the community relationships we form give us a sense of purpose and meaning that hugely impacts our health and longevity. Sometimes these cultural connections are found in large events that are planned throughout the year. Other times, we see how simply preparing and eating food together serves our need to strengthen our relationships with one another.

Just as the Standard American Diet (SAD) negatively impacts the diet component of the DRESS Code, so does the increasingly common way of American living pose an obstacle to our ability to foster strong communities with beneficial social ties. Research has shown that communities with a high number of fast-food restaurants, extraction industry jobs (mining, quarrying, oil and gas sectors), and high population densities have lower life expectancies. Again, the opposite is true. Communities like the Blue Zones, where people stick closer together on a social level, tend to enhance health and increase longevity.

A Word about Racism

The reality of systemic structural racism is another example of how our relationships affect our health. Racism is an affront to human dignity and a moral aberration that is ethically unacceptable. Furthermore, it is detrimental to our health and well-being on multiple levels. In fact, many cities, states, and nations have deemed racism itself to be a public health crisis. Racism negatively impacts how we relate to one another, with real-world consequences. Racism in its various forms has led to many tragic outcomes that have long gone unaddressed in our society.

Even more insidious and less clear to many is that the racism experienced on an almost daily level by individuals in the form of microaggressions directly impacts our health. A variety of studies have shown acts of discrimination to contribute to premature aging and chronically elevated stress hormones, resulting in increased risk for high blood pressure and metabolic diseases.

As discussed earlier, inflammation over time is an underlying factor for many diseases. In this case, chronic inflammation at the molecular level is likely responsible for the innumerable health stats, where Black and Brown Americans have poorer health outcomes for every major disease and longevity across the board compared to their White counterparts. This is a social justice *and* health issue for all those involved. Working to optimize health by enhancing our relationships must include addressing the persistent role of racism in our lives to allow all of us to achieve our true potential in all dimensions of life.

Spirituality and Health

Many cultural practices come from spiritual and religious traditions that have withstood the passage of time. Engagement in religious community life has also been shown to be a fruitful way to ensure meaningful relationships that enhance our health.

Historically, the connection between religion and medicine has been strong. Often physicians have been members of the clergy or healers in indigenous communities around the world. And some of the first hospitals were created and run by religious orders. It is fitting, therefore, to see how engagement in religious activity can benefit your health.

There is a growing body of research looking at the relationship between religion/spirituality and health, and showing that religion and spirituality help people deal with acute and chronic illnesses. A significant chunk of this research has looked at the impact on mental health. Spirituality has also been shown to increase positive emotions, such as hope, self-esteem, and meaning or purpose in life. Given these findings as related to mood, engagement in religion has also been shown to help with depression and anxiety.

Research also reveals that engagement in religious or spiritual activities can help prevent heart disease, the progression of certain cancers, and ensure mental health to avoid dementia. In fact, a growing body of literature has shown strong associations between attending religious services and longevity.

This research shows that attending faith-based services four times per month will add four to fourteen years of life expectancy.[26] One study found that women who went to any type of religious service more than once per week had a 33 percent lower chance of dying as compared to their secular peers over a sixteen-year follow-up period.[27] Another study found a link between attending religious services and reductions in our stress response (and therefore inflammation) and mortality, with those attending these activities being 55 percent less likely to die during the eighteen-year study than their non-religious peers.[28]

Many of these benefits tie into the idea that a community, or network of meaningful relationships, leads to epigenetic changes that increase health and longevity. Being a part of a community of believers also helps to reinforce healthier behaviors. In some cases, that is explicitly part of being a good member of that community. The Adventist community in Southern California is a great example of this. Adventists live longer and are healthier than their fellow Californians literally across the freeway. Their faith includes a dedicated day every week as time for reflection and connecting with family, as well as a plant-based diet without alcohol or tobacco use. Having these healthy norms as part of their faith community reinforces and strengthens the ability of this community to access the core elements of the DRESS Code and live healthier for longer.

Find a Furry Friend

While it is important for all of us to cultivate meaningful relationships with other humans, developing loving relationships with animals is also beneficial for our mental and physical health. Studies have shown that having pets can reduce stress, anxiety, and even ease feelings of depression and loneliness. Pet owners also tend to be more physically active (especially true for dog owners), which results in better fitness levels. The presence of any animal can significantly improve our blood pressure, resulting in lower risk for a heart attack or stroke.

Pets are also a vehicle through which we can connect with others. Think of a dog park where people come to socialize their dogs and also connect with one another. Some research has even shown that older adults have slower cognitive decline if they own a pet. One study found that older adults who owned a pet for more than five years were able to score higher on cognitive tests than those without pets. I find my own connection with my cats to be fulfilling every day when we spend quality time together, and this is true of countless others who cherish the animals in their lives.

How to Stay Connected

As we have seen, the R in the DRESS Code for relationships is quite important. As some researchers have described, the "social genome" is a concept that describes the impact that our relationships with one another have on our gene expression. As with the other DRESS Code epigenetic inputs, the quality of our relationships can directly impact the expression of our genes for better or worse.

- Social Genome/Quality of our Relationships à Gene expression modification (DNA Histone Modification or DNA Methylation or MiRNA changes) à Metabolic Changes in Physiology à Optimal Health Outcomes including Longevity and Wellbeing

The COVID-19 pandemic taught us that we can stay connected even while being physically distant from one another. Thanks to modern videoconferencing technology and smartphones, our dear friends and loved ones are simply a click away on a screen, where we can hear and see them live from anywhere in the world. The availability of this ability to connect virtually has allowed many businesses to continue their work remotely and contributed to the ongoing capacity for our world to remain productive during different points of the pandemic. However, even more important than ensuring commerce and work goals, the ability to connect is fundamental to achieving health and well-being on all levels.

The more connected you are with others, the less likely you are to have anxiety or depression. People who are more connected have greater self-esteem and empathy for others. They also show greater levels of trust and willingness to cooperate, leading to even greater points of connection and harmony in their relationships with others.

As there are thankfully many ways to stay connected and avoid the pitfalls of loneliness, we want to share some tips for staying connected.

First, remember that it is never too late to connect. Studies have shown that retired men who found new friends to replace work buddies were happier and less lonely. These friendships may not always be smooth or perfect, but the key is that you feel that you are not alone, and you have someone to turn to when things get tough.

People who are lonely often report missing simple things that can make a big difference to combat their isolation and loneliness. These include being in the presence of another person, laughing together, hugging, sharing a meal, going for a walk, traveling, or just holding hands. If you already have people in your life to do these things with, try to do some of these simple yet impactful things every day. If you are isolated and need to develop these important relationships, here are some important ways to get out there and reconnect with people:

- Join an in-person or online group that is aligned with your interests (a Meet Up group, a book club, a sports league).

- Reach out and touch someone—contact a friend and reconnect using the telephone or videoconferencing.

- If you are part of a religion or church, attend services and gatherings where you can meet and connect with fellow members of your community.

- Volunteer—sometimes doing service is the best way to meet like-minded people.

- Make a plan to get out there and out of your comfort zone in talking with others or prioritize the friends and relationships you already have in your life.
- When spending time with others, open up authentically about yourself and be an active listener.
- Be humorous; studies suggest that laughter and the use of humor brings us closer together.
- Lend a helping hand—research shows that both giving and receiving assistance can help us get closer with one another.
- Express gratitude—showing appreciation with specific points about another person that you value will help strengthen your bonds.
- Express affection—this can take many forms, from verbal to physical touch; the key here is to say how you feel.
- Move together—dancing or walking or doing any activity together that includes moving naturally is another way to connect.

CHAPTER 6

E IS FOR EXERCISE: WHEN IN DOUBT, JUST START MOVING

If exercise were a prescription medication that could be contained in a pill, it literally would be the most prescribed medication of all time. Exercise is the first and critical E of the DRESS Code. Like D for Diet, exercise is a key epigenetic input that updates our genetic software with far reaching implications for almost every part of our bodies. Let's start with some definitions.

Any movement that causes skeletal muscle contraction resulting in an increased energy expenditure from our normal resting state can be considered physical activity. Exercise is a special form of physical activity that is planned, structured, repetitive, and with the purpose of improving physical fitness, health, or performance. Although I will focus on the impact of exercise, any physical movement is beneficial for health. In fact, people in Blue Zones don't have an expensive gym membership or personal trainer; instead, they move naturally as part of their daily routine. Research has validated the fact that the risk of dying prematurely declines as people become more physically active. So movement is key.

As the law of physics states, a body in motion tends to stay in motion, while an object at rest tends to stay at rest. Movement is life—think of a moving stream of water. Stagnation is death—think of a puddle where there is no water flow. This scientific law helps to explain why physical activity is so important. Turns out, if you don't move it, you do lose it.

Exercise is beneficial because of its direct impact on gene expression. By changing the expression of our DNA at the molecular level, exercise can update our genetic software and enhance our health. Exercising regularly for even just six weeks can modify our risk for disease. Exercise results in improved muscle development and metabolism. The figure below illustrates the epigenetic pathway for exercise.

- Epigenetic Input: E for Exercise à Gene expression modification (Histone or Methylation) à Metabolic Changes in Physiology à Reduced/optimal weight, blood sugar, blood pressure, mental health, heart health, immunity, anti-aging impact on all cells and tissues/organs

Exercise involves movement, and this stresses the body while you are doing it. Unlike harmful kinds of stress, the stress from exercise is short-term and beneficial. An exercise routine that stresses our heart makes our heart stronger and healthier. Exercise empowers us to do more physically while decreasing our risk of a heart attack or stroke.

When You're Just Starting a Workout Routine

We've all experienced the soreness that comes from working out. When we first start exercising, our bodies hurt. This can be very discouraging, but it's actually a good sign. Although painful, it's beneficial to have a certain amount of soreness in our muscles in the beginning. This soreness is a result of exercise breaking down our muscles and then rebuilding them stronger than before. Too much of this can lead to injuries, but the right amount of exercise, starting low and increasing slowly, will lead to incremental improvement and success. Make sure to get plenty of rest between exercise sessions; this is what gives your body the time to recover and rebuild. And remember to drink lots of water—exercise increases our need for hydration.

What Happens When We Exercise?

When we first start to exercise, our body begins to make changes to keep up with the higher level of physical activity:

- Our heart and lungs begin to work more to continually provide adequate oxygen to our tissues, temporarily raising our heart rate and our blood pressure.

- Blood flow is redirected away from our digestive system and toward our skeletal muscles to keep us moving. (That's why it's not a good idea to exercise right after a meal when our body moves, blood flows to our digestive organs so we can effectively digest our food.

- Blood flow increases circulation throughout our bodies, healing our tissues and removing metabolic debris.

- Our brains produce serotonin, dopamine, and GABA, enhancing our experience and providing better brain function following exercise.

After an exercise session, our body compensates and "recovers" (returns to normal) by lowering our blood pressure and heart rate. Interestingly, our body doesn't simply go back to the same heart rate and blood pressure levels as before—instead, it goes even lower. This sustained heart rate and blood pressure-lowering effect is an important "side effect" that helps us stay healthy. That's why athletes have lower resting heart rates—exercise has made their hearts more efficient.

For the next several days after exercise, our metabolic rate is increased, making our metabolism faster and more efficient. At the cellular level, the powerhouse that produces our energy—the mitochondria in our cells—begins to multiply within days of exercising. This results in more energy production and translates to feeling more energetic. Mental changes also occur, boosting your mood within minutes of exercising with the release of endorphins, and this lasts for several days after your exercise session. All these changes make exercise an important therapy for high blood pressure, depression, and fatigue.

What Are the Benefits of Exercise?

One indicator of the benefit of physical activity is the impact of low cardiorespiratory fitness (the ability of our heart and lungs to deliver oxygen efficiently to our cells during physical activity) as a risk factor for premature death. Low cardiorespiratory fitness found in people who are inactive has been shown to be the leading cause of preventable deaths from all causes, more than obesity, smoking status, high blood pressure, cholesterol, or diabetes. In fact, the risk of dying prematurely from any cause declines as people become more physically active. This demonstrates how important it is for us to be physically active and consider engaging in some form of exercise.

There is specific strong evidence that physical activity lowers the rate of a number of conditions, including coronary heart disease, high blood pressure, metabolic syndrome, type 2 diabetes, breast cancer, colon cancer, depression, and even falling.

Exercise fundamentally changes gene expression to improve our health. For example, signal pathways that code for heart failure can literally be turned on by a sedentary lifestyle or turned off by regular physical activity. This and other epigenetic switches are responsible at the molecular level for the benefits of exercise.

Stress from high blood pressure makes us sick, while the stress of exercise keeps us healthy. (This is an example of unhealthy versus healthy stress, which I will discuss further in the next chapter on Stress.) With uncontrolled high blood pressure, there is no relief from the stress that is placed on the blood vessels and heart. This uninterrupted, constant stress turns on the switch for heart attacks and strokes, and eventually leads to heart failure.

In the case of exercise, however, the stress that leads to an elevated heart rate and blood pressure is temporary because we rest after our activity. This resting period gives our body the chance to recover and benefit from exercise. Our genetic software is updated, and the right metabolic pathways are created to sustain and strengthen our heart cells. This protects our heart and allows us to optimize heart function and longevity.

Physical activity strengthens our blood vessels and increases their lifespan by allowing them to remain elastic, not resistant and tensed. Our heart literally becomes stronger at the cellular level from exercise, while it withers and dies without it. In the past, patients who have had heart attacks were told to stay in bed and avoid any physical activity. This led to people dying from recurrent heart attacks. But now, a key part of recuperating from a heart attack is a comprehensive cardiac rehabilitation exercise program specifically designed to heal your heart after a heart attack or stroke and keep you from having another one.

The best treatment for most joint pains and muscle strains is exercise—specifically physical therapy. Although it may not seem intuitive, the targeted movements utilizing the injured joint are key to recovery and pain relief. For example, lower back pain is one of the most common reasons for a visit to the doctor's office. Every day millions of people sprain their lower back. Staying in bed and avoiding movement only makes it worse. Instead, if you walk gently and do lower back–stretching exercises, you will experience pain improvement and faster recovery. The same is true for mild ankle sprains or knee sprains. Even the symptoms and progression of arthritis can be markedly improved with specific exercises targeting the muscles that support your joints. For example, in many cases, knee arthritis symptoms and the need for surgery can be delayed or prevented completely by regular physical therapy exercises.

Exercise also strengthens your lungs. Regular exercise expands your lung capacity, making this organ stronger, as your muscles get stronger. As your fitness level improves, your body becomes increasingly more efficient at delivering oxygen to the blood and transporting it to all your cells. This is one main reason people who exercise regularly do not get short of breath as easily as people who are out of shape. Regular exercise like swimming or yoga that incorporates rhythmic breathing can further strengthen the ability of your lungs to maximize their ability to inhale oxygen and exhale toxins with every breath.

Exercise also boosts our mood by releasing endorphins that result in a "contact high," where we experience feelings of joy and happiness simply by engaging in this activity. The powerful impact of exercise on mental health has been shown to be equal to standard antidepressant medications in treating mild-to-moderate depression.[29] In fact, in the UK and other countries, a diagnosis of mild-to-moderate depression triggers an exercise prescription (in addition to therapy and meditation) prior to considering prescription drugs.

In addition to improving the function of our heart, lungs and muscular systems, exercise can enhance brain health, decreasing the risk of cognitive decline, memory loss, and certain forms of dementia. Research has shown that regular aerobic or cardiovascular activity, the kind that gets your heart rate up, boosts the size of your hippocampus, the part of the brain important for memory and learning. Other research shows that exercise can even reverse mild cognitive impairment (difficulty with thinking and memory) in the early stages. These findings suggest that exercise can be an important tool for combating dementia, a national pandemic where one person is diagnosed every four seconds!

Exercise's impact on memory is multifaceted. Exercise improves our mood and our ability to sleep, and it reduces stress and anxiety—all of which contribute to the chronic inflammation that leads to cognitive decline. Exercise also reduces insulin resistance, a key cause of type 2 diabetes. The inflammation resulting from insulin resistance can stimulate the release of factors or chemicals in the brain that reduce the ability of brain cells to grow and survive. In fact, several studies have shown that people who exercise have higher brain volumes and, therefore, healthier function in the prefrontal and medial temporal cortices, the parts of the brain that control thinking and memory.

Exercise boosts our immunity. That's right, exercise can even increase the ability of our immune system to fight off infections. As blood flow increases and circulation improves, our immune cells also circulate more freely throughout the body, making them more effective in recognizing potential harmful viruses or bacteria and neutralizing them before they have a chance to take hold. The activity of our immune cells is also enhanced, as exercise enables the cells to do their job more efficiently and effectively. Physical inactivity has the opposite effect. As with the other epigenetic switches, we can upgrade or downgrade our genetic software through what we do or don't do.

Complementing the R in the DRESS Code—relationships and social connection—exercising together is also beneficial. Connecting with others as workout buddies or teammates in sports not only provides the physical benefits of exercise, but also has the bonus of building relationships.

Where Do I Start?

First of all, any movement or physical activity is better than nothing. Research shows that the biggest impact is seen from the first phases of activity. In other words, when you go from no activity to walking for fifteen minutes a day, there is a huge positive health impact associated with this. So, the truth is any movement will have a benefit.

Let's say you aren't physically active. Your starting point may only be to reach 50 percent of your maximum heart rate, working your way up gradually. The best first step is to begin with walking. Walking alone works wonders. For those who are living a sedentary lifestyle, walking alone for as little as twenty minutes a day can decrease the risk of a heart attack by 30 percent, without any other lifestyle changes!

Exercise can be categorized into four major types: aerobic, strength training, stretching, and neuromuscular. There are benefits from each of these types of exercise, so balancing each of them into your weekly regimen is a good long-term goal. Aerobic activity improves the body's composition and cardio-respiratory fitness level. Examples of aerobic exercise include walking, jogging, bicycling, using a treadmill, or dancing to Zumba. Muscle-strengthening exercise increases muscle mass and improve endurance. Some examples of muscle-strengthening include lifting weights or doing push-ups and pull-ups. Stretching exercises like yoga or lower back stretches provide flexibility and relief of muscle tightness to prevent injury. Activities such as tai chi increase balance, agility, and proprioception (your body's ability to sense movement, action, and location, thus preventing falls).

Aerobic exercise can be light, moderate, or vigorous. Aerobic exercise is the best type of exercise for heart health. Its benefits include lowering bad cholesterol and raising good cholesterol, lowering blood pressure, and helping with weight loss. You can assess the benefits of aerobic exercise by checking your heart rate and symptoms of breathlessness. For someone who is not active, simply walking up a flight of stairs can raise their heart rate to high levels and result in shortness of breath. The same flight of stairs may not raise heart rate or cause any shortness of breath in someone who is fit.

Based on the evidence for how much aerobic exercise is needed to get the most impact, the recommendations are 150 minutes of moderate intensity aerobic activity or 75 minutes of vigorous-intensity aerobic activity. This can be spread out in shorter intervals, such as twenty or thirty minutes, multiple times throughout the week. The best way to determine if your activity is moderate or vigorous is by the Talk Test. If you can talk and sing easily while exercising, then you are only doing light-intensity exercise. If you can easily talk but not sing while you are doing your activity, then you are doing moderate intensity. If it is difficult to even talk a few words without pausing for a breath during the exercise, then you are doing vigorous activity.

One of the best ways to assess your cardiorespiratory fitness is to do a VO2 max test that measures how much oxygen you consume while exercising. This is typically done with a treadmill or bike and equipment that analyzes the air you exhale to assess your body's oxygen consumption.

Going from a deconditioned state to a fit state takes time. The body needs to adapt to the changes with cycles of intensity/stress and calmness/rest. Remember, if you push yourself to do too much too soon, you can injure yourself and do more harm than good. In general, once you start, do the same routine (frequency, intensity, and duration) for the first two weeks before increasing any part of it. If the same activity no longer causes your heart rate to go up as high and you recover more quickly during rest periods, you know you have improved your fitness, and you can add a little more to your regimen. Building incrementally will result in great success.

When it comes to strength training exercises, it's all about the amount of resistance and the repetition of the activity. It's also about which muscles are exercised. The goal here is to do muscle-strengthening activity at least two days a week. Over the course of a week, you want to rotate through all upper and lower body muscles, including a concentration on your core.

Whether you are using weights or resistance bands or doing push-ups and using your own body and gravity, heavier loads with lower reps is a key part of developing strength. If the goal is endurance, then lighter loads with increased reps are needed. Usually, weight loads between eight to fifteen reps will facilitate both muscle-strengthening on the lower end and endurance on the high end.

Start with lighter weights with lower intensity and increase slowly. This can include increasing the number of reps you do for a given activity, shorter periods of rest between reps, or increasing the frequency of resistance exercise sessions. To master a certain level, it's better to increase your reps before increasing your load. When the same weight or level or resistance does not require as much strain, then you know you have built muscle and can push yourself a bit further to the next level.

Exercises such as yoga or simple stretches help to develop balance and flexibility. When targeting specific issues like lower back pain, daily stretches can help by preventing lower back strain—the most common cause of lower back pain. A good time for stretching is during the warm-up phase of an exercise session, and again as part of a cool-down routine. Stretching has many surprising health benefits. Any soreness you may feel for several days after the workout is a sign that it is working. Remember, all exercise affects your muscle, breaks it down at the molecular level, and turns on genes to repair it. That's why having periods of rest is so important for the magic of exercise to happen at the cellular level. A good rule of thumb is to add an extra thirty minutes of sleep at night after you have started to work out or had a particularly intense workout session.

Warmup—Stretches followed by resistance
muscle-strengthening exercises
Conditioning—Aerobic exercise, preferably HIIT
Cool Down—Muscle-strengthening/resistance and stretching

You can expect to progress through three major phases when you start an exercise program:

1. Initial conditioning: You begin to establish new routines of activity with cycles of rest.

2. Building momentum: This usually starts after several weeks of consistent low-level activity.

3. Maintenance: This phase is both simple and challenging; it involves maintaining the new level of fitness you have achieved and sticking to your routine.

Stop Sitting Around

Most people spend approximately eight to ten hours a day sitting. A recent meta-analysis of multiple studies has shown that prolonged sitting disrupts metabolic health. Even after just thirty minutes of sitting, blood flow decreases, muscles become less responsive to insulin, and our uptake of glucose slows down. All this leads to higher blood sugar and insulin resistance, which increases our risk for type 2 diabetes and poorer circulation, which increases risk for stroke and higher triglycerides. The key is to break up sitting time as much as possible to improve blood flow and increase skeletal muscle activation. I recommend interrupting sitting every fifteen to thirty minutes with short bursts of activity, such as walking or doing squats.

HIIT It!

High-intensity interval training (HIIT) refers to a specific type of aerobic exercise. The basic idea is to have a short cycle of intense exercise, then rest. You exercise intensely for two to three minutes, and then take two to three minutes to rest or exercise much less intensely. For example, on a treadmill, you can speed up for two minutes, then slow down for two minutes. This oscillation between increased and decreased speed or elevation on a treadmill has remarkable benefits for your heart and blood vessels. While higher levels of activity can be achieved during the intense periods for those who are more fit, even small levels of intensity can be powerful when practiced with resting intervals in between. And it's *never* too late for HIIT. One study of heart failure patients found HIIT for thirty minutes three times a week for thirty days literally reversed the severity of their heart failure—and in some cases reversed it completely![30]

Rest Is Important

It appears that the rest period between exercise sessions is the key feature that makes it healthy, as opposed to chronic stress, which leads to unhealthy inflammation and disease. Without rest, only damage can occur. That's why long periods of high-intensity workouts can do more harm than good. When we exercise too intensely without adequate rest for recovery and repair, there is no time for our software to update itself. Instead, we get the coding that leads to further damage and disease, thus losing the potential benefits of exercise. Too much high-intensity exercise without adequate time for recovery generates disease-causing free radicals and damages our hearts and bodies. The more free radicals we have, the faster we age. That's why the antioxidants found in plant foods are so beneficial—they reduce inflammation and neutralize free radicals. Exercise can also enhance the production and effectiveness of antioxidants if done in moderation with adequate rest intervals. Getting adequate rest between workouts for optimal recovery is just as important as the exercise session itself.

What If I Have Been Diagnosed with Heart Failure or a Debilitating Condition?

One landmark exercise study included patients diagnosed with heart failure (stages 2-4). Each stage of heart failure is associated with poorer heart function and the ability to be physically active. In the study, the heart failure patients in various stages were asked to engage in HIIT at their level of ability for thirty minutes three times a week for four weeks. After four weeks, the patients who were stage 3 or 4 became stage 2 or 3, and many of the those who were stage 1 or 2 reversed their heart failure without any additional medications. This demonstrates how powerful exercise can be, even when we are seemingly on our last leg.

All You Have to Do Is START

The DIY part of all this is the most exciting part of the DRESS Code. You don't need expensive equipment or to hire an expensive professional to get started. The DIY concept applies to the E in the DRESS Code, just like all the other letters. YOU have the power to change your genes, update your software, and achieve optimal health and longevity.

With any lifestyle change, people are often overwhelmed by the gap between where they currently are and where they want to be. We might be too intimidated to start, and so we keep waiting for the perfect moment—or we try to do too much too quickly; we can become a weekend warrior and injure ourselves, leading to a setback and recovery. Or we may not be able to achieve what we set out to do, and in our disappointment, we give up too quickly.

Starting with a small, easily accomplished goal builds momentum and ultimately leads to success in establishing new healthy habits. The way to do this is to just START. This can be as easy as picking out a first step—for instance, going for a walk. This first step needs to be specific and time bound. In other words, when will you walk and for how long? "I will walk for fifteen minutes three days out of the next seven days on Monday, Wednesday, and Friday from 5:30 p.m. to 5:45 p.m., when I come home from work."

Now, you are ready to achieve it.

Check to see if this seems achievable first. If your confidence level in accomplishing a goal is greater than 7 out of 10 (with 10 being 100 percent), you will likely do it. If you can't honestly give it a 7 or greater, try doing less. Maybe you decide to do two fifteen-minute sessions in the next week. Then see how you did at the end of the week. If you did your two fifteen-minute sessions, great—now it's time to repeat it! There's no need to jump too quickly into doing more; instead, establish this as a new, healthy habit. After your body and brain adapt to this, you'll be ready to add another session or more time, etc. This approach really works. I've seen it succeed with our patients, and even with ourselves.

Here are some additional ways to make exercise a part of your life:

- When in doubt, just move. Remember, any natural movement and physical activity will deliver health benefits.
- Set a reminder to stand or move every thirty minutes.
- Take a five-minute walk after meals.
- Do body-weight exercises (squats, lunges, calf raises) when taking breaks from sitting.
- Try using a standing or treadmill desk while you work.
- Take walking meetings on the phone instead of sitting in front of the computer.

- Walk or pace back and forth while watching TV instead of sitting.

- Use a pedometer or wearable device to track your physical activity level. For some of us, seeing the numbers and where we fall short motivates us to stay engaged.

- Find a workout buddy. Having an accountability partner for exercise ensures you make it to the gym or do that scheduled workout instead of blowing it off.

- If you can, hire a personal trainer. Not everyone can afford this option, but for those who can, paying someone motivates you to get your money's worth to follow through and get it done.

- Invest in a gym membership or home gym equipment. Whether it is a treadmill, exercise bands, or weights, having the tools you need in the convenience of your home makes it easier to commit to a regular exercise routine.

- Make a commitment. Just like any goal in life, exercising requires commitment. Decide to make it a priority, add it to your calendar, and engage your partner and family to hold you accountable to follow through on your commitment.

- Look for additional resources online. We've included a resources list with helpful links at the back of the book.

Remember, exercise doesn't have to be in a gym or with high-tech equipment. Turning on the music and dancing by yourself or doing housework, like mopping your floor, raking leaves, or anything that gets you moving, counts! So, "wax on, wax off" to get the benefits of exercise anywhere, anytime.

CHAPTER 7

S IS FOR STRESS: OVERCOME ADVERSITY AND BUILD RESILIENCE

Stress: The Good and the Bad

Stress is the first S in the DRESS Code, and it has a far-reaching impact on our lives. Like all other DRESS Code elements, stress can have a positive or negative impact on the development of disease or the expansion and establishment of health. Without stress, we cannot get the edge we need to meet the deadlines and challenges of the moment. Short-term stress, like acute inflammation, can be quite beneficial and even essential for achieving our goals in life.

However, also like chronic inflammation, stress over time can negatively impact every system and part of our bodies. In this chapter, we explore what stress is and how it can be both good and bad. We discuss how stress can downgrade or upgrade our genetic software, depending on the kind of stress and its timing. The way we choose to view each stressor in turn affects whether we can successfully cope with it. We look at how resilience and grit can help us adapt to stress in a healthy manner.

In 1936, Hans Selye defined *stress* as "the non-specific response of the body to any demand for change."[31] This definition emerged from Dr. Selye's research on animals, where he noticed how disease developed not just from known disease-causing factors (e.g., low-fiber diet with high red meat consumption and colon cancer), but also from the impacts of negative stress. The concept of stress historically focused on the negative aspect of stress, with standard dictionaries defining it as "physical, mental, or emotional strain or tension" or "a condition or feeling experienced when a person perceives that demands exceed the personal and social resources the individual is able to mobilize."

Although this definition makes all stress negative, stress can either be good or bad. In fact, Selye defined good stress, or eustress, as the form of stress that resulted in better outcomes, including health and success in life. For example, the stress experienced by an athlete in a race is eustress; the pressure exerted on the person makes them stronger to win the race. Although this can be unsettling, imagine a blacksmith forging a metal sword in the heat of the hearth, continuously hammering on the anvil and shaping the metal until all the edges are perfect. The creation of a finely tempered sword out of a raw piece of metal is like an individual's transformation into an athlete from repeated positive stress that remakes them into a high-performing superstar. This is a great way to think about how stress can result in optimal health.

Elasticity, a concept from physics, also fits within this picture. Elasticity is the ability of a material to resume its original shape and size even after being compressed or stretched out by an external force or stressor. This scientific concept parallels the concept of grit or resilience, our ability to cope with the stressors we experience in life. This ability to cope and adapt determines our ultimate success or failure in dealing with stress.

This is a good time to call out the health benefits of activities that put stress on our bodies in a healthy way. Physical activity and exercise are great examples of activities that exert healthy stress on our bodies. As discussed in the previous chapter, the stress of exercise on our bodies temporarily raises our blood pressure and heart rate. Once our session is over, there is a prolonged blood pressure lowering effect.

Over time, maintaining cardiorespiratory fitness through regular activity that positively stresses our bodies results in more efficient and healthy heart function. It also keeps our arteries elastic and flexible, preventing our blood pressure from rising and increasing our risk for heart disease or stroke.

Another example of good stress for our body is spending time in a sauna. Saunas have been used for hundreds, if not thousands, of years in some form. Where I live in Arizona, one indigenous tradition is the "sweat lodge," which is a sauna-like setting where people gather. In this case, this practice has been a part of a culture and spiritual tradition. In other parts of the world, like Northern Europe, wood-based dry saunas are routinely visited multiple times per week.

Research has shown that exposure to high heat in a sauna is beneficial. These benefits include lower blood pressure, improved pain relief from arthritis, improved skin health, reduced negative stress and chronic inflammation, and boosted immunity. In a twenty-year Finnish study with two thousand people, those who used a sauna two to three times per week had a 24 percent lower risk of death, while those who went four to seven times a week had a 40 percent reduction in death compared to those who went for just one session a week.

The typical time spent in a sauna can be anywhere from five to twenty minutes, but studies have shown that those who spend twenty minutes versus ten minutes have a 52 percent lower risk of heart-related death.

One of the reasons for these health benefits is that the stress of exposure to high temperatures over short periods of time mimics the effects of exercise on our bodies. In the same way as exercise raises our heart rate and blood pressure temporarily, a short time in a sauna does the same thing.

Sauna, steam room, hot tub, and other heat therapies work by increasing the production of heat shock proteins (HSPs). HSPs help other proteins to refold in a way that prevents them from being damaged, which happens over time as part of aging or exposure to chronic inflammation (from chronic negative stress).

In the case of damaged proteins, HSPs help to break these down and recycle them so the damaged proteins do not accumulate. Additionally, HSPs activate other repair mechanisms that ramp up internal antioxidants to protect us from oxidative stress (the stuff of aging at the molecular level, which I will discuss in detail in chapter 9). HSPs also reduce AGEs, which are the inflammatory products formed from too much sugar binding to proteins and damaging them. Other benefits of heat therapy include maintaining insulin sensitivity, improved sleep, and reduction of stress hormones throughout the body.

Now, I would not try this without talking to your doctor first, and when you do begin, it is important to make sure to be hydrated before, during, and after. Even five minutes in a sauna can be beneficial, and you can gradually work your way up to longer periods (not to exceed twenty minutes).

Just as the stress of higher temperatures has benefits, so too does the stress of lower temperatures, such as doing a cold-water plunge or immersion. The stress on our bodies for this short time results in long-term benefits, including improved mood through the release of endorphins and dopamine; reduced inflammation by constriction of blood vessels; reduced muscle soreness, especially from exercise; boosted immune function; improved sleep quality, improved cognitive function; activation of brown fat, which can help with fat burning and optimizing weight; and boosted metabolism.

Going back and forth between hot and cold waters can also have its benefits. The stress of both improves circulation of blood and lymph (immune cells) throughout our body. This helps to clean out toxins more efficiently and prevent infections more effectively by having our immune cells disbursed throughout our body. The same benefits as listed above from the heat and cold therapy can also be experienced here.

The timing of stress plays a role in whether the stress is beneficial or detrimental, and the amount of stress is also proportional to the impact it has on us. As noted with heat and cold therapy, these are recurrent short bursts of exposure to the stress of higher or lower temperatures. Similarly, as seen in the curve below, the initial mental stress we experience can be quite useful for enhancing our performance. Think of times when you have to make a presentation in front of a group or are facing a demanding day at work. Experiencing stress in these situations pushes you to do your best; this stress only improves your abilities and hones your strengths.

Our Response to Stress

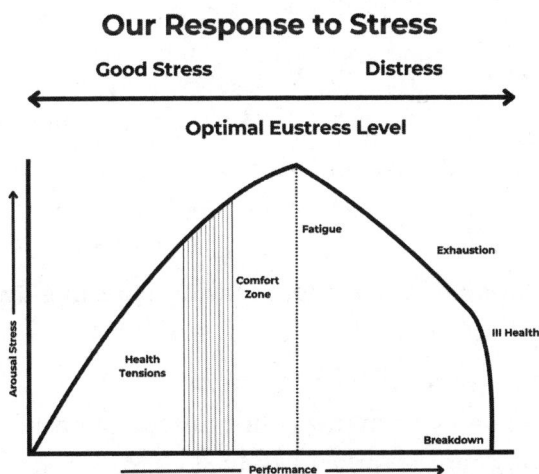

Human Response to Stress Curve Adaptation of the Yerkes-Dodson Human Performance (*according to Nixon P: Practitioner 1979, Yerkes RM, Dodson JD) Creative Common Copyright found in Rapolienė L, Razbadauskas A, Jurgelėnas A -Advances in preventive medicine(2015) online at https://openi.nlm.nih.gov/ detailedresult?img=PMC4383502_APM2015-749417.001&req=4

Another example might be a chronic procrastinator—the stress of a deadline improves the ability to focus and accomplish tasks. I have tapped into the power of this good stress a few too many times. These are all examples of good stress, just like good acute inflammation is a key part of healing.

At some point, however, if you experience stress for too long without rest and recovery, you will get to a tipping point, where the good stress becomes bad. Past a certain point, there are diminishing returns, and more stress results in the worst outcomes. Chronic stress, like chronic inflammation, then becomes the negative DRESS Code input, leading to downgraded genetic software and disease. This is the bad side of the stress coin. Our bodies and minds begin to break down with increasing wear and tear, leading to depression, exhaustion, and eventually disease.

The American Psychological Association broadly categorizes stress into three major groups: acute, episodic acute, and chronic.

- **Acute stress** is the initial response to an emergent situation, such as a noise, danger, a deadline, or upcoming performance.

- **Episodic acute stress** refers to an intermediate level of stress where someone's life is overly demanding or chaotic. This is found more commonly in people who overcommit, spreading themselves too thin and constantly feeling the pressure of having to catch up.

- **Chronic stress** can be both internal and external. Externally, this stress may form from unhealthy relationships at work or at home, financial difficulties, the loss of a loved one, and other major life events. Internally, the way we cope with these, and other types of stress, determines how we can thrive despite them. Negative self-talk and being overly critical only make this type of stress worse, dampening our ability to stay positive. This leads to negative health consequences.

How Common Is Stress?

According to the American Psychological Association (APA), stress is all too common and was worsened by the COVID-19 pandemic in 2020 and 2021. Prior to the pandemic, the APA conducted a national survey. In their 2021 report, Stress in America,[32] *they assessed the impact and status of stress in the United States. Some key findings included the following:*

◊ *More than three-quarters of adults report physical or emotional symptoms of stress, such as headache, feeling tired, or changes in sleeping habits.*

◊ *44 percent of adults say they exercise or walk to manage stress, and 47 percent say they listen to music. More than one-third (37 percent) spend time with friends or family.*

◊ *Nearly half of adults say they have lain awake at night because of stress in the prior month.*

◊ *Nearly three in five adults say they could have used more emotional support in the last year.*

How Do I Know If I Am Experiencing Negative Stress?

Negative or chronic stress can occur from a variety of sources. These can include troubled marriages or relationships, conflicts at work, or financial difficulties. Signs of stress can be physical, emotional, psychological, or behavioral.

Signs of Stress

- Difficulty concentrating, worrying, anxiety, and trouble remembering
- Easily angered, irritated, moody, or frustrated

- Changes in appetite, including emotional eating, changes in sexual drive, abnormal periods or changes to the normal cycle, high blood pressure, frequent sore throats and colds, headaches and fatigue, and weight gain
- Unhealthy relationship with drugs, such as alcohol, inadequate self-care and declining hygiene, feeling of powerlessness, signs of depression

The Impact of Stress on Our Bodies

When we are acutely stressed, our bodies enter what is known as the "fight-or-flight" state. In this state, physiological changes happen to prepare us to engage an external force or stressor. This state is thought to be a part of the evolutionary process dating back to the time when we faced predators, such as lions in the wild. In those moments, we had to be able to either fight or take flight to survive. This is now understood as part of the autonomic nervous system, the part of our nervous system most sensitive to stress, both good and bad. It is generally broken into two major components: sympathetic or parasympathetic.

The sympathetic nervous system is activated during times of arousal or excitement. In modern life, this may be right before a meeting, or in a social gathering, or any other activity when there is great anticipation or anxiety. In those types of situations, the sympathetic nervous system goes into full effect, increasing our heart rate and blood pressure, giving us sweaty palms, dilating our pupils to take in our surroundings, and diverting blood flow to our skeletal muscles. We might experience an immediate energy boost. Within the first minutes to hours of a stress response, our immune system is enhanced and functions better than normal. Short-term stress also enhances both memory formation and memory retrieval. All these helpful tools give us that short-term burst to perform and address the urgent matter at hand.

For short-term performance needs, this acute stress response is beneficial. But when persisting long term, these same changes can be destructive. Chronic stress has been linked to an increased risk of high blood pressure and heart disease, including higher rates of heart attacks and strokes. Constantly mobilizing materials (amino acids, glucose, and fatty acids) for a fight-or-flight attack is inefficient. Over time, this can lead to a form of insulin resistance (the underlying cause of type 2 diabetes) that is stress-induced. Long-term stress over weeks, months, and years can inhibit our immune system, as well as our body's ability to prevent the development of autoimmune diseases and certain cancers.

In terms of brain health, long-term stress impairs our memory. This directly acts on the hippocampus, leading it to shrivel up, atrophy, and retract a bit. Memories become more difficult to access. Persistent chronic stress can lead to several psychological and physical symptoms, such as headaches, fatigue, upset stomach, changes in weight, anger, anxiety, depression, and difficulty sleeping.

Chronic stress impacts all major systems in our bodies and has been linked to impaired immune function, decreased bone density, problems with memory, weight, abdominal fat deposition, insulin resistance, high cholesterol, increased risk for blood clots, impaired wound healing, poor sleep, and even decreased longevity through shortening of telomeres (more on this marker for aging in Chapter 9).

HOW STRESS AFFECTS THE BODY

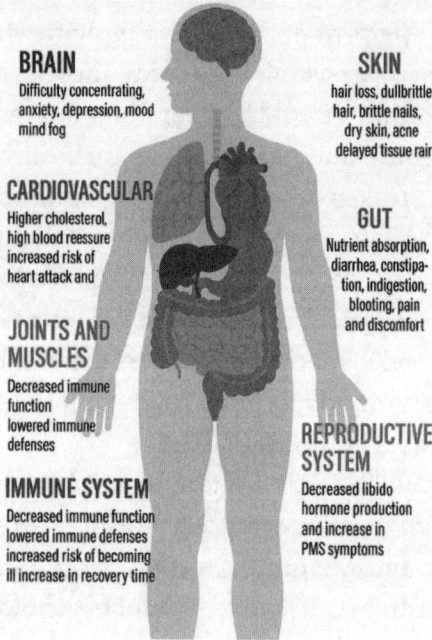

BRAIN
Difficulty concentrating, anxiety, depression, mood mind fog

SKIN
hair loss, dullbrittle hair, brittle nails, dry skin, acne delayed tissue rair

CARDIOVASCULAR
Higher cholesterol, high blood reessure increased risk of heart attack and

GUT
Nutrient absorption, diarrhea, constipation, indigestion, blooting, pain and discomfort

JOINTS AND MUSCLES
Decreased immune function lowered immune defenses

REPRODUCTIVE SYSTEM
Decreased libido hormone production and increase in PMS symptoms

IMMUNE SYSTEM
Decreased immune function lowered immune defenses increased risk of becoming ill increase in recovery time

People who have chronic stress also tend to adopt unhealthy habits, such as smoking, physical inactivity, poor dietary choices, and heavy alcohol use.

Stress as an Epigenetic Input

So, what happens to our genes when we experience stress? In acute stress, our genes respond to urgent needs by altering their expression to address the acute stressor in a timely and efficient matter. The physiological adaptation to stress is known as allostasis. This term basically describes the process of changes in gene expression and physiology to cope with an acute stressor. In the short term, this can occur swiftly and effectively to gear up and then gear down after the stress has been resolved. The problem occurs when the stress continues; our ability to cope over time weakens. The changes in gene expression go from being a natural response to an unhealthy state of stress overload. During persistent chronic stress, our genetic software is downgraded, and we have a decreased ability to cope with the stress. The key point here is that the type and timing of the stress determine the impact of the stress as either a good or bad thing.

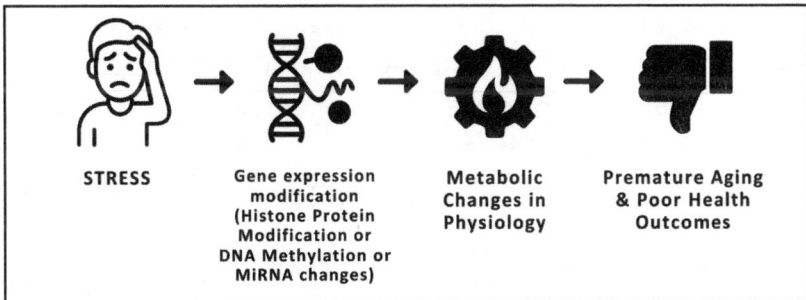

STRESS → Gene expression modification (Histone Protein Modification or DNA Methylation or MiRNA changes) → Metabolic Changes in Physiology → Premature Aging & Poor Health Outcomes

Where we live, our work, our relationships, what kind of food we have access to, our economic status, and our mental health all affect our ability to cope with stress. If a family is experiencing food insecurity, there is a stress associated with that. If a person loses their job or has problems at work, this can be another source of stress. All of these factors can impact our mental health and result in changes in our gene expression.

For example, persistent financial hardship has been linked to changes in gene expression that are directly tied to depression. This same gene change occurs in children who experience adverse childhood experiences (ACEs). These potentially traumatic experiences occur between birth to age seventeen, and may include violence, neglect, abuse, and substance-abusing parents or caregivers. These events and other forms of trauma at any point in life can result in changes in gene expression, leading to an increased risk for chronic diseases, including depression, PTSD, anxiety, diabetes, heart disease, cancer, obesity, and lack of overall well-being.

Research has even shown that having six or more ACEs in life shortens one's lifespan by as much as twenty years. Given such a lasting impact, all efforts aimed to address and prevent such traumas are critical.

How to Cope and Overcome Chronic Stress

Thankfully, there are many ways to manage stress and develop resilience to overcome life's many challenges. If you have experienced trauma or other difficult circumstances, you might want to consider asking your primary care physician for a referral to therapy and counseling. Today, many forms of therapy are highly effective for processing and dealing with chronic stress. In addition, the following key strategies can help.

The Relaxation Response

Picture this: You have just finished a delicious, nourishing dinner. It's winter, and you are sitting by the fireplace on your favorite couch. You are reading an enjoyable book or watching your favorite show. Your blood flow switches from your skeletal muscles to your intestines to enable you to fully digest your meal. Your brain waves shift to patterns associated with calmness, and you generally feel a sense of comfort and relaxation.

But you don't need all of that to get to this state. The Relaxation Response, a term coined by Harvard researcher Herbert Benson, uses meditation, breathing, or simply reframing the way we think and experience things around us to achieve a state of deep relaxation while being awake. Mindfulness, Transcendental Meditation, or simply focusing on your breathing in a comfortable, quiet space all help elicit this response. There are even smartphone apps to help you meditate to get into the zone of relaxation. Meditation is effective in helping lower blood pressure, decrease anxiety, improve depression, assist with insomnia, help with chronic pain, and even help improve brain health. This is really a "choose your own adventure" experience, so approach it with an open mind and realize there's no wrong way of doing it, as long as you are putting in effort to get into that relaxed space.

One easy way to do this is to focus on our breath. Breathing is a unique activity, as there are both conscious and unconscious elements involved. Often, we do not think about breathing as it just happens. Our brain helps to ensure this steady and continuous flow of life-giving oxygen and life-affirming exhalation of toxins with CO_2. Other times, we can choose to hold our breath. Breathing has been a part of meditative practices for thousands of years. Unfortunately, our modern life has made our breathing problematic, which diminishes our ability to cope with stress.

Optimal breathing can enhance our health and our resilience. A key component of optimal breathing is deep breathing. Deep breathing can improve our digestion by "massaging" our abdominal organs. It can also help to ensure optimal immune function by improving blood and lymph circulation (lymph circulation is the movement of immune cells throughout our body that allows them to find potential pathogens and neutralize them before we get sick).

Deep breathing also results in more signals sent through the vagus nerve, which elicits the Relaxation Response. This can help to lower cortisol (stress) hormones, blood pressure, and improve markers of heart health. The best way to breathe more deeply is to engage in "belly" breathing. I learned to do this in high school when I was in choir and served as a vocalist in the performing arts. Singers need to take good, deep breaths from their belly to maximize their voice.

But don't worry, you don't need to be a trained vocalist to take advantage of this skill. To do this, simply place your hand on your belly and take a deep breath, pushing your belly out against your hand. This is the best way to breathe, as our diaphragm flattens down to expand our lungs, resulting in a smooth "massage" of all of our abdominal organs below it. Shallow breathing involves using our shoulders and rib cage; this is not healthy and is actually a sign of lung disease. Training ourselves to breathe more deeply is a great way to reduce stress.

Another way to optimize our breath is to slow the pace of breathing. Deeper breaths that are slower are better. Breathing more quickly is less efficient, as we only end up using half the air that we have potential access to. What is healthier is to breathe more deeply and slowly, so you can use more of the air with life-giving oxygen.

Instead of breathing twelve to eighteen breaths per minute, optimal deep and slow breathing should put you between eight to twelve breaths per minute. Research in rhythmic breathing cycles in Buddhist monks has been shown to lower heart rate (making the heart a more efficient pump), increase oxygen to the brain, reduce anxiety, improve memory, and shift the body into a more parasympathetic, relaxed state. But again, you don't have to be a monk to do this. Simple breathing exercises can help you train your lungs to breathe more slowly and deeply.

My mentor, Dr. Andrew Weil, often speaks about the 4-7-8 breath, which helps elicit a relaxed state: Inhale for 4 seconds, hold for 7 seconds, then exhale for 8 seconds. Another option is to take three slow breaths as you push out your belly and flatten your diaphragm, then exhale slowly for 8 seconds through pursed lips. In all instances, it is best to breathe in from your nose. Breathing in from the nose is important, as the nasal passages are filled with small hairs that act like filters to filter out potential toxins and germs from the air. Breathing from the nose also results in 18 percent more oxygen than breathing in from the mouth.

Studies have shown that mindfulness-based stress reduction (MBSR) can change the structure and function of key areas of our brain that help with our response to acute stressors. The eight-week course in MBSR originally developed by Dr. Jon Kabat-Zin is now available online from many organizations. The goal of this course is to integrate mindfulness into daily living and apply it to mental and physical challenges that life brings.

Participation in this eight-week course has been shown to increase thickness in the prefrontal cortex, the part of the brain that helps us with reasoning or rational thought and decision-making. It also results in an increase in gray matter density in the hippocampus, a key area of the brain responsible for learning, new memory formation, emotional regulation, and self-awareness. Additionally, there is a decrease in gray matter density in the amygdala in just eight weeks. The amygdala is often referred to as part of the "reptilian brain." This is the emotional part of the brain that has a very knee-jerk response to things based on emotions.

Take the example of getting cut off by another driver in traffic— the amygdala is the part of the brain that sets off your tendency to yell or curse or, even worse, try to cut them off. Reducing gray matter in the amygdala is associated with reduced stress, anxiety, and negative thoughts. Decreased brain matter in the amygdala, along with increased thickening in the other areas (prefrontal cortex and hippocampus) from mindfulness meditation practice, results in an improved ability for us to deal with negative stressors. Studies have confirmed that MBSR has had a number of specific benefits, including enhanced psychological hardiness (or resilience, as we will discuss later), lasting decreases in physical and psychological symptoms from illness; improved chronic pain, anxiety, depression; and the development of compassion and empathy for the self and others. This is a powerful tool that can help us act instead of react to such situations.

Additionally, ancient cultural and spiritual practices can help elicit a relaxation response and mitigate the impact of chronic stress, while also connecting individuals with a higher sense of purpose and meaning. These practices collectively have been referred to as mind-body therapies and include daily activities such as yoga or tai chi. Engaging in these helps develop resilience in the face of adversity and stress. They can dramatically improve our ability to deal with stress when it happens, and reframe it in a way that is understandable and manageable. Both tai chi and yoga, for example, have a long list of health benefits, including:

- reducing stress, anxiety, and depression
- improving sleep
- treating addiction
- preventing falls
- reducing the risk of heart attacks
- lowering blood pressure
- boosting immunity
- improving muscle strength and flexibility
- managing diabetes
- aiding rehabilitation after stroke
- helping with chronic fatigue syndrome

Yoga and tai chi classes are now widely available in many parts of the United States and around the world. Additionally, online videos exist to demonstrate how to do it, so learning these healing practices is easier than it ever has been to experience.

Other ways to manage chronic stress is self-expression, which can take many forms. This can include journaling, as well as engaging in some form of artistic expression, like painting or sculpting, playing a musical instrument, singing, or dancing. Reading a book or listening to music are other simple coping mechanisms for stress. Getting a massage is another experience that can help relieve stress. As noted in the chapter on Relationships, connecting with others can help with stress relief through the support that comes with community. This can include quality time with family or friends, as well as spiritual or religious activities.

Coping with Negative Stress and Resilience

How we cope with or adapt to stressors in life makes a huge difference in the relative impact of stress on our well-being and health. Having a sense of control, the confidence to believe in ourselves, and the social support to enhance coping skills determine how well we ultimately process trauma and the resulting chronic stress that comes into our lives. The famous psychiatrist and Holocaust survivor Victor Frankl is widely quoted as saying:

> Between stimulus and response, there is a space. In that space is our power to choose our response. In our response lies our growth and our freedom.

This concept formed the core of Frankl's psychotherapy, known as logotherapy. How we choose to view stressors like divorce, death, or financial ruin is something no one can control. Our perspective forms in that space between the stressor and how we choose to respond. Understanding that the choice ultimately is ours is key to understanding how to positively cope with negative stress.

Our power and freedom is the ability to choose how to interpret what we have experienced and what to do with the time that has been given to us in life. How we perceive life—whether we see the glass as half full or half empty—is critical to managing stress, overcoming challenges, and achieving mental health and well-being. Frankl's book *Man's Search for Meaning* details his experience in Nazi Germany's concentration camps and provides the essence of his approach to psychotherapy. Basically, Frankl observed that what differentiated those with the mental and emotional strength to survive the inhumane and horrific concentration camps was a sense of meaning and purpose.

In contrast to Sigmund Freud, Frankl believed that our ultimate search as humans was not for pleasure, but for meaning and purpose. Therefore, logotherapy helps patients find a sense of meaning and purpose, which helps them overcome mental illness and achieve their goals. You don't have to have a mental illness to benefit from this form of therapy. The idea is to find what gives you a sense of purpose or meaning, and use that as a source of motivation for you to find health and happiness.

The importance of meaning and purpose in life is one of the key characteristics of people who live in the Blue Zones. In the Costa Rica Blue Zone, it is known as *plan de vida*, or "life plan or purpose," while in Okinawa, Japan, it is referred to as *Ikigai*, or "discovering what worthy gifts you have to contribute to the world with your life." In the Adventist community in Loma Linda, California, the believers are called to a sense of purpose as a part of their faith, which gives meaning to their actions and goals.

Discovering your passion and purpose in life is something that is specific to you. It is empowering to know that it has so many benefits, giving us the resilience we need to face life's challenges and stressors.

> *Our greatest glory is not in never falling but in rising every time we fall.* —*Confucius*

Speaking of resilience, this quote captures the essence of resilience. As challenges arrive for all of us, we experience stress. Over time, this can result in chronic stress. Instead of negative thinking focused on failure, which can make us even less hopeful and worsen our negative stress, we can choose to see failure as an opportunity to learn and grow. That way, any failure we experience in life is an opportunity to learn and grow, an opportunity to get us closer to our goals and achieving success. In essence, we must learn to fail well to live well and be well. This is the key to resilience.

Psychologists define resilience as the process of adapting well in the face of adversity, trauma, tragedy, threats, or significant sources of stress—such as family and relationship problems, serious health problems, or workplace and financial stressors. As much as resilience involves "bouncing back" from these difficult experiences, it can also lead to profound personal growth. It's our capacity to bounce back—not what happens, but how we choose to act when things happen—that defines us and our resilience. Resilience, therefore, is a key part of overcoming stressors in life to stay healthy.

One way to think about this is to understand that all dimensions of life include some form of resilience. For example, physical resilience (perhaps most intuitive) can be seen in an athlete's ability to maintain endurance and physical prowess despite higher-than-normal physical demands and stressors.

Like physical resilience, emotional resilience involves flexibility and regulation (the stuff of emotional intelligence) to adapt to changing and unforeseen circumstances in life. Cultivating resilience in the different aspects of life is a good practice for all of us to optimize our ability to combat the effects of chronic stress.

Here are some key points to consider for building resilience:

- Accept that change is inevitable, and realize that life never stays the same, so however bad things seem, they will not last forever.

- Reframe how you think about stress; accept that it is inevitable, but use it to grow and learn, rather than as an excuse to be sad or give up.

- Develop an internal locus of control; realize that your perception controls the impact stress has on you, not the stress itself.

- When you encounter challenges, recognize it's a specific issue that can be addressed, not a global problem with everything in life.

Another important way to cope with stress is to tap into another DRESS Code element: Relationships. How much social support we have in the form of meaningful, authentic relationships can markedly enhance our ability to mitigate the impact of stress on our lives. Investing in these important relationships—not just superficial friends on social media, but genuine, lasting friendships—can improve our ability to cope with the changes and chances that occur in our lives.

CHAPTER 8

S IS FOR SLEEP: DREAM OF A HEALTHIER, HAPPIER YOU

Sleep is as ancient as life itself. Some version of sleep takes place in virtually every form of life on this planet. Whether it is a period of dormancy and regeneration for single-cell organisms or complex patterns of sleep phases in mammals, every living thing sleeps.

Scientists continue to debate the main purpose of sleep, but one thing is clear: Sleep is an essential part of life. Without adequate quantity and quality of sleep, we are exposed to short-term and long-term threats to our health and survival. Sleep impacts almost every aspect of our function as human beings. Sleep determines physical and mental health, as well as our ability to be creative and learn. Therefore, the second S in the DRESS Code is Sleep.

There are several major theories for why we sleep. One theory is based on the evolutionary benefits of being inactive at night. This theory suggests that animals that were able to stay still at night had an advantage over animals that remained active. Through natural selection, these animals did not get killed by predators or have as many accidents while being awake at night.

Another major theory for why we sleep is that of energy conservation. This suggests that the primary purpose of sleep is to reduce our individual energy demand to require less food to survive. In support of this theory, energy metabolism is reduced by 10 percent in humans and more in other species during sleep. Both caloric demand and core temperature also decrease during sleep. This is part of the story, but certainly not all of it when understanding why we sleep.

Another long-standing theory with a large body of evidence to support it suggests that sleep restores what we have lost while awake and provides an opportunity for our body to repair itself. Much of the health benefits of sleep and the dangers of inadequate sleep point to the reality of this theory. Many of the body's major repair functions occur during sleep, some of them exclusively. Critical functions include muscle growth, tissue repair, protein synthesis, and growth hormone release.

Sleep also impacts our cognitive function. For example, the chemical substance adenosine is a by-product of active neurons engaged in thinking and daytime activities. A buildup of adenosine leads us to feel tired, which, in turn, triggers sleep. During sleep, the body clears adenosine from our brains and systems, leading to a feeling of alertness when we wake up. Caffeine blocks the action of adenosine, giving us an alert feeling, but not actually getting rid of adenosine. This gives us a false sense of energy despite not having had enough sleep. We usually need eight hours of sleep to fully purge our brains of adenosine buildup, which is why getting less sleep results in us feeling more tired.

Sleep is also linked to brain plasticity—the ability of our brain to grow and create new neurons. Scientists have only recently realized that brain plasticity is not limited to childhood but can occur at any age. Yet the role of sleep in the growth of new neurons is particularly critical in childhood, when infants spend thirteen to fourteen hours a day sleeping.

Sleep plays a role in memory by activating the hippocampus, the part of our brain that concerns emotions and memory. Sleep is an important part of learning and maintaining working memory in life. Sleep also enhances the parts of the brain that regulate our emotions, including the amygdala, striatum, hippocampus, insula, and medial prefrontal cortex.

For instance, when we have adequate sleep, our amygdala is less active (similarly to those of us who do the MBSR course). Therefore, we are able to respond in a more nuanced and adaptive way to acute stressors. When we are sleep-deprived, our amygdala is hyperactive, making us more susceptible to emotional deregulation and overreacting to acute stressors, which can make our lives even more stressful.

Clearly the main purpose of sleep is the role it plays in regeneration, restoration, repair, and health maintenance. Sleep impacts virtually every system of the body. Before we dive deeper into the impact of sleep on human health, let's discuss what sleep is.

What Is Sleep?

Now that we have explored why we sleep, let's understand what sleep is and how it impacts us. Sleep is essentially the opposite of wakefulness. It is a special state of being in which our cognitive functions are not turned off but rather switched from external to internal mode. Many systems shut down, while others ramp up. Our brain wave patterns change when we enter sleep.

In humans, sleep consists of two major brain wave patterns: non-rapid eye movement (NREM) sleep and rapid eye movement (REM) sleep. The biggest contrast in brain wave patterns occurs during NREM sleep. When we are awake, we have rapid brain wave patterns. During NREM, our brain waves are ten times slower than when we are awake. During this phase of sleep, our brain's logic center (cortex) is completely relaxed, and our external-facing senses are dormant. Our brain shifts short-term memories from the front of the brain into our long-term memory bank in the back of the brain. The next phase of sleep is REM sleep, when our brain waves become rapid again. This is the phase of sleep when we most commonly dream. In REM sleep, we experience feelings and see our life passing by with different images and sensations as our eyes move rapidly while closed.

When we are awake, we get all sorts of inputs that impact us. We learn in school and in life. We make connections and conclusions based on our observations. We experience joy and pain. In NREM sleep, our bodies store these experiences as data points and individual skill sets. REM sleep takes things to the next level by integrating and connecting them to make sense of it all as part of a complete picture of how life works.

REM sleep allows us to develop new perspectives and insights that enable us to engage in critical thinking and problem-solving. There are a total of four phases of sleep: the first three are NREM, and the fourth and final phase is REM. Each sleep cycle lasts between seventy to 120 minutes on average.

Virtually every body system changes during the shift from wakefulness to sleep. During sleep, our breathing follows the pattern of our brain waves, slowing down during NREM sleep and then becoming irregular and more rapid during REM sleep. Our heart rate also follows a similar pattern. Our muscles relax during NREM sleep as our total energy expenditure drops. During REM sleep, our muscles are atonic, or paralyzed. This seems to be a protective mechanism to prevent our limbs from moving during the dreams we experience in REM sleep.

Our hormonal patterns also change during sleep in accordance with our body's internal clock (known as the circadian rhythm). Melatonin, a key hormone for sleep, increases as we approach the time to sleep; this helps us wind down and get ready to fall asleep. Once asleep, the growth hormone surges, which helps us grow when we are younger. This is one reason we need more sleep during childhood. In adults, the growth hormone supports a healthy metabolism and the continued maintenance of bone and muscle integrity and cellular mechanisms that prevent premature aging.

Cortisol, or the stress hormone, which is a key part of waking up in the morning and having the energy to get started with your day, decreases during the first few hours of sleep. You will recall that chronic elevation in cortisol leads to chronic disease. Sleep is the original stress reliever, as it helps our body relax and lower these inflammatory hormones. During sleep, our immune system releases cytokines, chemical messenger signals that also fight off inflammation, treat underlying infections or trauma, and boost immune function. This includes the body's surveillance work that finds precancer cells and destroys them before they lead to cancer.

The Impact of Sleep on Gene Expression

Having adequate quality and quantity of sleep directly upgrades our genetic software. Having inadequate sleep downgrades our genetic software. In this way, sleep or the lack of sleep works like the other DRESS Code inputs on our genes.

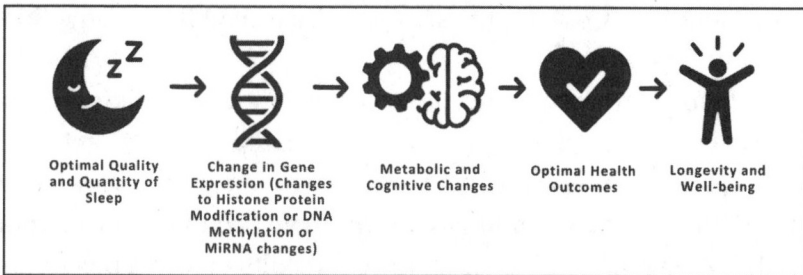

| Optimal Quality and Quantity of Sleep | Change in Gene Expression (Changes to Histone Protein Modification or DNA Methylation or MiRNA changes) | Metabolic and Cognitive Changes | Optimal Health Outcomes | Longevity and Well-being |

Recent research has shown that sleep directly changes our gene expression for better or for worse. Our lifestyle can lead to sleep deprivation. Working longer hours, taking stimulants like coffee to stay awake, and exposing ourselves to excess light at night are all contributing factors. This leads to increased inflammation and stress hormone activation. These pathways result in changes in gene expression that are directly associated with inadequate sleep. These changes in gene expression result in memory problems, difficulty in thinking, an impaired ability to focus, and less creativity. Metabolic changes (insulin resistance, weight gain, high blood pressure) also occur, leading to disease.

There is a bidirectional relationship between stress and sleep. Both are key DRESS Code inputs that can lead to health or disease. How we cope with stress and how we protect our sleep impact each other, resulting in wellness or illness. Stress regulation is associated with changes in gene expression (REF 8.8). Our ability to cope with stress results in upgraded genes, while inability to cope results in chronic stress.

Excess chronic stress leads to changes in our brain's hippocampus, resulting in poorer sleep. The hippocampus is the portion of our brain that is involved in memory and learning. Poorer sleep increases our stress response. The process by which this happens is again through changes in our DNA software, for better or for worse. Chronic sleep deprivation leads to these changes in our genes that also worsen our ability to cope and adapt to chronic stress. All DRESS Code inputs are related, as we will see in the final chapter of this book.

Chronic inflammation increases our risk for certain cancers, cardiovascular disease, diabetes, and obesity. Sleep deprivation leaves us susceptible to infections and even developing cancer. Low levels of melatonin, a key hormone for sleep, have been linked to tumor growth. More exposure to light at night results in lower melatonin levels, and our genetic software is downgraded, allowing tumors to grow freely.

The Impact of Sleep on Health and Disease

Sleep impacts almost all aspects of our health, whether mental, emotional, or physical. As mentioned, the most compelling purpose for sleep involves restoration and repair. Without this time to repair, damages at the cellular level will lead to chronic inflammatory changes and disease. A major cause of chronic inflammation for many of us is sleep deprivation. Inadequate or poor-quality sleep can damage almost every system of our body, leading to premature disease and premature death. On the other hand, good, adequate amounts of sleep result in a symphony of hormonal changes and almost musical interactions that keep our bodies healthy and balanced throughout the cycle of life. This fine-tuned ensemble of hormonal shifts with sleep has implications for inflammation and our ability to repair and regenerate every night to start fresh the next day.

Not getting enough sleep also disrupts our sex hormones, resulting in reduced sex drive and less interest in sex. In fact, men who suffer from sleep apnea have been found to have lower testosterone levels, and regular sleep disruption can also impact fertility by reducing the secretion of fertility hormones in women.

Studies have shown that people who sleep less than seven hours a day tend to gain more weight and have an increased risk for obesity compared to those who get at least seven hours of sleep each night. Additionally, eating more at night contributes to weight gain and weight retention, as compared to eating during the day, when we are more active and can burn those calories. Sleep deprivation may be linked to an increased risk of obesity, metabolic syndrome, and type 2 diabetes.

There is also a direct link between heart health and sleep. Getting less than seven hours of sleep a night leads to elevated risk factors for heart disease and metabolic syndrome. Inadequate sleep has also been linked to calcification of our coronary arteries, another known risk factor for a heart attack. These risk factors include high blood pressure, insulin resistance, weight gain, chronic inflammation, and increased cortisol levels.

Each additional hour of sleep over five hours per twenty-four hours decreases blood pressure. In fact, most people with high blood pressure will benefit from adequate sleep as a key part of their treatment plan.

One of my patients, Jennifer, came to me with a new diagnosis of high blood pressure. At the time, Jennifer was in her late thirties. When seeing anyone with high blood pressure, I always ask about each of the DRESS Code elements. In Jennifer's case, her diet was mostly plant-based with no processed food, she was married and had a great relationship with her husband, was physically active, with regular exercise sessions of over 150 minutes of moderate activity weekly, and had a good support system that helped her to manage her stress.

Unfortunately, Jennifer was not sleeping well. Between work and her two young children, Jennifer was sleeping an average of only four to five hours a night. We discussed how sleep could play a role in her high blood pressure, and I spoke with both her and her husband about realigning their schedules and support to ensure that Jennifer could sleep more.

It wasn't easy, but after a couple weeks of making adjustments, Jennifer began routinely sleeping six hours a night, and after a couple of months, she was able to get to at least seven hours of sleep. All along I had asked her to monitor her blood pressure, and we saw it come down as her sleep increased. Although I had initially started Jennifer on a low-dose blood pressure medication, after addressing her sleep, we were able to wean her off the medication completely, and her blood pressure remained normal.

Sleep also helps maintain brain health. Benefits of adequate quality sleep include improved memory and improved creativity in approaching our daily tasks. Lack of sleep has been associated with memory problems and premature aging of the brain. Lack of sleep can also impair our ability to focus and concentrate on our work. Sleep deprivation has, moreover, been linked to a variety of mental health disorders and even to the development of Alzheimer's disease.

How Much Sleep Do We Need?

Achieving optimal sleep is about both quality and quantity. A minimum seven hours of sleep for adults is required, while eight is considered optimal by many sleep experts. According to the Centers for Disease Control (CDC), each age group has a different sleep requirement, as the following table shows.

That's why their sleep patterns are rather erratic before this rhythm is established.

Newborn	0–3 months	14–17 hours (National Sleep Foundation) No recommendation (American Academy of Sleep Medicine)
Infant	4–12 months	12–16 hours per 24 hours (including naps)
Toddler	1–2 years	11–14 hours per 24 hours (including naps)
Preschool	3–5 years	10–13 hours per 24 hours (including naps)
School Age	6–12 years	9–12 hours per 24 hours
Teen	13–18 years	8–10 hours per 24 hours
Adult	18–60 years	7 or more hours per night
	61–64 years	7–9 hours
	65 years and older	7–8 hours

Some sleep experts argue that we should aim for at least eight hours of sleep after age eighteen. Obviously, sleep needs will vary depending on underlying medical conditions, stressors, and level of daily activity. Students may need more sleep to consolidate all the knowledge they are learning every day. Someone who is physically active and exercising more will require more sleep on those more intense workout days for muscle recovery and buildup. In general, for adults, getting seven to nine hours of quality sleep per night is a great goal to work toward.

How Much Sleep Are We Getting?

Despite the clear benefits of sleep and the need for adequate quality sleep, our modern life—with bright lights at night, chronic stressors, and the use of caffeine to burn the midnight oil—has led to an epidemic of sleep deprivation.

According to the CDC, 70 million Americans have chronic sleep problems, and one in three adults don't get enough sleep. A global sleep survey in 2019 showed 62 percent of adults report they don't sleep as well as they would like. Insufficient sleep may be more chronic for some, but one CDC study showed that as many as 70 percent of adults report they have insufficient sleep at least one night a month. Sleep disorders, like chronic diseases, are more common in underserved populations and Black and Brown communities.

Unfortunately, the odds of being sleep deprived have only increased in the last thirty years (CMOS), leading to more than an estimated $100 billion in lost productivity, sick leave, medical expenses, property and environmental damage. Lack of sleep is such a big problem that the CDC declared sleep deprivation to be an epidemic.[33]

The same states with extensive sleep deprivation also have higher levels of obesity, diabetes, and heart disease. All these conditions are linked together in part due to sleep and in part due to the other elements of the DRESS Code. How we live, including how much sleep we get, impacts our genetic software for better or for worse.

How Do We Improve Sleep to Heal and Live Optimally?

The balance between sleep and wakefulness is part of a larger rhythm of life. Most living creatures have an internal clock based on a twenty-four-hour day. This internal clock, or circadian rhythm, helps to regulate our sleep schedule, appetite, body temperature, hormone levels, daily performance, blood pressure, and mental health. Disruptions of the rhythm can occur in people who travel extensively and experience jet lag and in shift workers who work night shifts.

Increased chronic stress and a lifestyle that includes erratic hours can also disrupt this rhythm and, consequently, impact our ability to achieve optimal sleep. Our sleep schedule is impacted by how we live every day. The more consistent our schedules are, the more success we have not only with sleep but with all the other DRESS Code inputs.

Consistency in our schedules helps our bodies gear up for life's daily activities and wind down for sleep. Take, for example, the rumbling you feel in your stomach when it is time for lunch. That sensation is actually your pancreas releasing all the enzymes needed to digest a full meal before you have even taken your first bite. If we eat at the same times, are physically active at the same time, sleep at the same times, and even have bowel movements at the same time, we will live a healthier and longer life.

While we need new information and challenges to stimulate our brains every day, we need regularity in terms of these essential life activities for our bodies to optimize their function. The sleep cycle fits well with this, which is why one key way to address insomnia is to start by setting a consistent sleep and wake-up time. It is not helpful to spend too much time in bed when not asleep. In fact, most experts suggest limiting what we do in the bedroom to sleep and intimacy with our partners.

When it comes to sleep, our exposure to light makes a big difference. Exposure to sunlight earlier in the day helps to ensure rhythmic changes in levels of hormones, including melatonin, the sleep-inducing hormone. One strategy to improve sleep is to make sure to get plenty of natural light earlier in the day and then avoid excess screen time and bright light exposure in the early evening. You can also wear protective blue-light glasses at night.

As with breathing in general, breathing in through the nose is a key part of optimal sleep. A number of people with sleep apnea have difficulty breathing through their nose. It is a good idea to get this checked out if this applies to you. Emerging research suggests that mouth breathers snore more and have more potential events during sleep that result in lowered oxygen levels, which, over time, can contribute to various conditions like dementia.

One trend that is currently being studied is mouth-taping to ensure that we breathe through our nose and not through our mouth. While the evidence is still not substantial, mouth-taping may be a good way to help develop the habit of breathing through the nose to reduce snoring and optimize oxygen while we sleep.

Healthy practices like these are all part of good sleep hygiene. Some of the key components of sleep hygiene include the following:

- Committing to a consistent sleep schedule; sleeping and waking up at the same time every day
- Early daytime exposure to natural light
- Avoiding excess caffeine, especially in the afternoon or evening
- Staying hydrated during the day and avoiding excess water at bedtime
- Avoiding alcohol close to bedtime (this disrupts REM sleep and causes you to wake up throughout the night)
- Exercising during the day, not in the evening
- Eating dinner before 8 p.m. and avoiding late-night meals
- Avoiding napping for longer than twenty minutes, if you nap at all
- Creating a bedtime routine to signal your brain that sleep is imminent

- Dimming the lights about two hours before bedtime
- Avoiding stimulating activities for thirty to forty-five minutes before bedtime: screen time, checking emails, social media
- Creating a relaxing bedroom environment for sleep and intimacy (blackout curtains, white noise machine, cool temperature)
- Consider wearing blue-light blocking glasses at night to reduce blue-light suppression of melatonin levels, especially important if exposed to screens such as computer or phone.

Do Sleep Aids Work?

Sleep aids in the form of medication can help with sleep, but they are not a long-term solution. Like most medications, these do not come without side effects. I recommend making the changes outlined in this chapter to get off these medications. One of the safer and healthier options for sleep aid that I routinely recommend to my patients is magnesium glycinate. This form of magnesium can help with anxiety and sleep. I usually recommend patients taking this about thirty minutes before sleep. You can start with a dosage of 150 mg and go up to 300 mg if needed. Magnesium is an example of a mineral that our bodies need for many functions, so taking this for sleep has a number of benefits. However, I would not do this without first making the changes discussed here.

One patient came to me with insomnia. Jim had tried all sorts of medications for this but was worried about becoming addicted to them, not to mention the side effects. As all DRESS Code elements are connected, I asked him about each of these in his life. Jim told me that he would eat late dinners and often wake up with indigestion at night. I talked to him about shifting the timing of his meals to eat less and eat earlier.

Additionally, Jim would fall asleep watching television on the couch and then get up and go to bed in the middle of the night. We discussed better ways of sleeping—including sleep hygiene, which involves routines and practices to prepare for bed. I advised Jim to have a set bedtime and to get ready for bed thirty minutes prior to this. We discussed reading a book in bed instead of watching TV (bedtime reading has been shown to help with sleep).

As Jim made these changes, he was able to wean himself off of the sleep medications and also improve the quality and quantity of his sleep. As a positive side effect of this, he lost about twenty pounds from not eating at night, and his borderline high blood pressure was completely normalized as well.

Making simple changes to your habits related to sleep as experienced by Jennifer and Jim and countless others is something we can all do. It is much easier than you may think to identify the triggers for sleep deprivation and make some adjustments that will result in great improvement.

PART III

Applying the DRESS Code to Your Life

CHAPTER 9

AGE WELL WITH THE DRESS CODE

How is age defined? Is it just a number? Is it how old you feel or is it determined by when you were born? Some say aging is a state of mind and you're only as old as you feel. Aging can be experienced in different ways in all the dimensions of life: physically, intellectually, socially, or spiritually. In all these areas, aging is inevitable, and it is also relative. It can be rapid, or it can be slow.

In my clinical practice, I can tell you that not all fifty-year-olds look the same. Some look like they could be much older, and others look significantly younger. This difference is not just skin deep either. Laboratory studies, precision medicine tools, and innovative new tests reveal the impact of aging within. We can literally "look in" to see the difference in the age of organs such as the liver or the amount of visceral fat present in the belly. We all want to optimize our aging to stay healthy longer, look younger, and feel the best we can. As we learned earlier in this book, how we choose to live our life and the experiences we have are more critical to the way we age than our genes or our preset biology.

While it's true that aging and disease are both inevitable, when and how we get sick and how fast we age are not predetermined by our genes. It's how we live that determines the course and duration of our lives. It is not a matter of genetics, but rather of epigenetics—the key elements of our lifestyle that can either upgrade or downgrade our genetic software for better or worse.

This is the essence of the DRESS Code: The way we live can literally change the expression of our genes for better or for worse. How we eat, the relationships we have, how physically active we are, how we perceive and experience chronic stress, and the quality and quantity of our sleep all work together to shape the pace and quality of our aging. That these factors are almost entirely under our control is incredibly empowering. We can choose the path to healthier aging and a better healthspan.

The goal of longevity and prevention is to live *better* for *longer*. It's about experiencing health and wellness with a high quality of life for as long as possible. Being technically alive is not something any of us should strive for. While the average life expectancy has increased from forty-seven to around seventy-seven in the last hundred years in most developed nations, just living longer is not necessarily a great thing. Being alive with debilitating chronic diseases is a miserable experience.

Dan Buettner's work in discovering the lessons of the Blue Zones is particularly important. In the Blue Zones, people not only live longer, but they also live better with a markedly reduced burden of illness from chronic diseases. The lessons learned from the Blue Zones have reframed our thinking about aging. Instead of an inevitable decline, we can look at aging as a process that can be cultivated to expand our years of high-quality life without debility and disease. To understand how to achieve this, we must examine what aging looks like at the cellular level.

Aging at the Cellular Level

Each cell in our body has twenty-three pairs of chromosomes. Our entire genetic material lives on these twenty-three chromosomes. In fact, you may recall from your high school biology class that every time our cells divide through the process of mitosis, our chromosomes are copied and divide with them. The end of each chromosome is made of repetitive sequences of non-coding DNA called telomeres. These end segments, which resemble little hats on the ends of each chromosome, are like protective caps that preserve the chromosome from damage. They are a critical part of ensuring the safety of our genetic material during the process of new cells forming through mitosis.

Over time, our cells divide millions of times, and each time a cell divides, the telomeres become shorter. The shortening of telomeres is a result of both the division process and the level of oxidative stress in our bodies. You can think of oxidative stress as essentially metabolic "wear and tear" at the cellular level that damages our cells and accelerates aging.

The level of oxidative stress is directly related to the lifestyle choices we make and the level of inflammation in our bodies. As oxidative stress increases and damage occurs, telomeres become shorter and shorter. Eventually, the telomeres become so short that the cell can no longer divide safely. This is the molecular process of aging.

For example, animals with longer lifespans have a significantly slower rate of telomere shortening compared to animals with shorter lifespans. In addition to being a marker for aging, shorter telomere lengths have also been associated with a variety of preventable medical conditions, including many forms of cancer, stroke, heart disease, vascular dementia, obesity, diabetes, osteoporosis, and even wrinkles.

TELOMERE

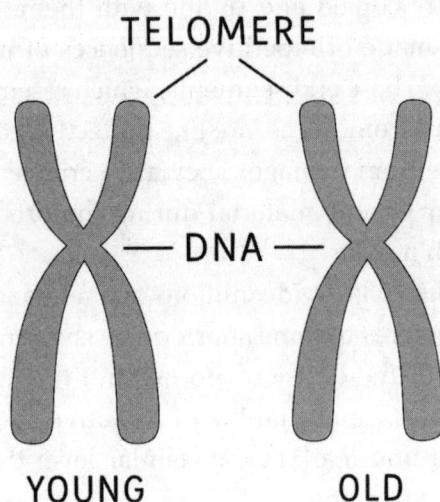

YOUNG   OLD

Research has shown a variety of interesting findings with respect to telomeres and aging. If we can slow down the shortening process or even lengthen telomeres, we can slow down or reverse the process of aging at the intracellular level. In fact, studies have shown that longer telomeres are associated with fewer illnesses and a longer life.

Aging and the DRESS Code

Let's examine how we use the DRESS Code to alter the course of aging and optimize our healthspan. One landmark pilot study conducted at UCSF followed thirty-five men with early-stage prostate cancer to explore the impact of lifestyle changes on telomere length, cancer progression, and health.[34]

The study included all the major DRESS Code elements except sleep. The men followed a diet of whole foods—plant-based and low in fat and refined carbohydrates. Participants walked thirty minutes every day six days a week. They managed stress by engaging in yoga-based stretching, breath work, or meditation for one hour every day. They also attended weekly support groups to connect with one another. These sessions included training on managing stress as well as counseling and some moderate exercise.

When compared to the group of twenty-five men in the matched control group, the group making these DRESS Code lifestyle changes demonstrated a significant 10 percent increase in telomere length! When the five-year study ended, the group that did not engage in these key lifestyle elements experienced a 3 percent shortening of their telomere length.

A recent study conducted by my longtime mentor and friend Christopher Gardner at the Stanford Prevention Research Center demonstrates how quickly and effectively diet can improve our health at the molecular level. This twins study is now featured in a Netflix documentary entitled *You Are What You Eat* and shows that a whole food, plant-based diet improved key health markers and increased telomere length in just eight weeks.

Beyond these studies, a growing body of research has already shown the impact of all the DRESS Code elements on telomere length and aging. For example, exercise has been associated with reduced oxidative stress and improved telomere stability and length. Athletes maintain longer telomere lengths over time, demonstrating a slower rate of aging at the cellular level.

Diets higher in whole, plant-based foods and fiber have been directly linked to reduced oxidative stress, which, in turn, improves telomere shortening. Limiting calories and protein from animal sources has also been directly linked to increased lifespan. The quality of our sleep and the duration of our sleep are both associated with metabolic age and telomere length.

Chronic stress also increases the pace of telomere shortening. People with untreated chronic pain and the high stress associated with it also have shorter telomeres compared to people without chronic pain and chronic stress. All the elements of stress discussed in the Stress chapter, including work-related exhaustion and negative stress, have been associated with telomere length. The greater the negative stress, the shorter the telomere length and the faster the pace of shortening. The reverse can also be true, as reducing stress and managing it through meditation or yoga or MBSR can help to slow down or even reverse the telomere shortening process.

Our relationships are also a key part of longevity. Older people with strong social support networks through meaningful, authentic relationships have longer telomeres. Married couples tend to have similar telomere lengths, demonstrating the impact of healthy or unhealthy behaviors on each other. Relationships should ideally reinforce healthy behaviors. And again, this can be synergistic in terms of DRESS Code inputs.

How to Reframe Your Life with the DRESS Code

While none of us can change our chronological age, our biological age is in our hands. Our future selves depend on the choices we make today in each of the DRESS Code lifestyle elements. As illustrated in this diagram, healthspan and longevity are directly impacted by each of the DRESS Code elements. Each element is like a double-sided coin.

For example, on one side, our diet can upgrade our genetic software, leading to optimal health and longevity. On the other side, a poor diet can literally turn on bad genes and downgrade our software. This is one reason dietary risk factors are now the number one risk factor around the world for premature, preventable death. We can literally turn this around by changing our diet. In the United States, we must change it by 180 degrees from the Standard American Diet (SAD). The double-sided coin of exercise versus a lack of exercise results similarly in health or disease, and so on for all the DRESS Code elements.

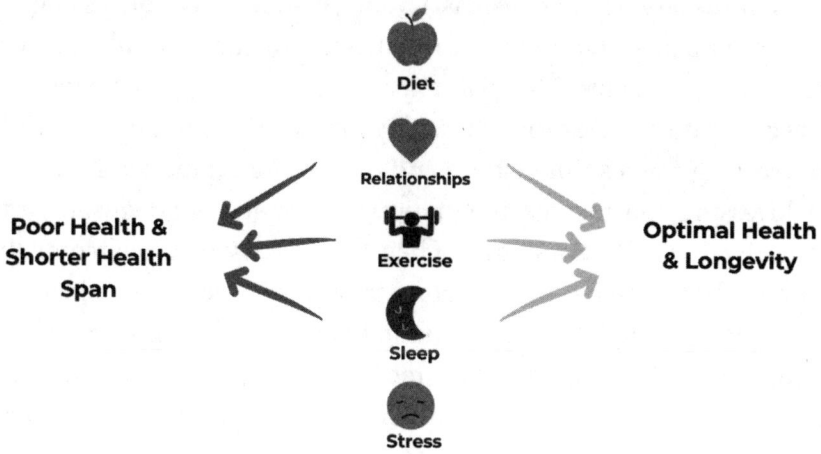

Recognizing the role the DRESS Code plays in determining our healthspan has many implications. There are a number of society-level changes that can set us up for success rather than failure.

Cutting physical education and what was formerly home economics programs from schools has resulted in generations of inactive people who don't know how to cook a healthy meal at home. While home economics was traditionally a women's subject, it really should not be defined by antiquated gender roles and instead be a universal part of primary education. Knowing how to prepare and cook real food is a life skill that allows us to optimize the D (for Diet) in the DRESS Code for a healthy life.

Having a food system that uses tax dollars to make processed foods cheap and widely available must change. Our tax dollars should be redirected to make real, healthy food inexpensive and accessible to all. Even the car-centered way of living in which we come back to our garages without connecting with others undermines our ability to create and cultivate healthy relationships in our communities. Shifting city designs to a town center with walking paths and services accessible through mass transportation would allow us to connect better with one another. This is happening in some of the more traditional Blue Zones around the world.

In a society where racism is a public health crisis, addressing the root causes of systemic structural racism to achieve health equity is critically important. This will expand the healthspan of people in the communities disproportionately impacted by this, by hopefully decreasing the resulting stress and chronic inflammation involved. Addressing the income inequality that creates food deserts and negative social determinants of health is necessary to overcome the impact that these have on chronic stress over time. Income inequality is also a public health crisis that sets us up for failure, where people have to work two to three jobs just to survive, a scenario that results in higher stress, poorer sleep, poorer diet, and greater social isolation.

All these public health and social justice issues are related to the DRESS Code. Addressing them on a societal level and addressing the DRESS code in our personal lives are important next steps in recognizing the role these elements play in our lives.

On an individual level, recognizing where and how the DRESS Code can impact health is critical to preventing, treating, and reversing the diseases of our time. The key is for all the elements to be addressed, not just one or two of them. Some of us may be great at exercising, but we never get enough sleep and are constantly stressed by unresolved issues at work and at home. Others may eat the best diet, but they never seem to lose weight because we do not get enough quality sleep and are physically inactive.

We are reminded of the many commercials for medications on television. One shows a man at a fair who tells his wife he would love to eat a hot dog, but he can't because of the indigestion it gives him. His wife smiles and tells him not to worry, all he needs is this little purple pill, and he can eat the hot dog without any problems! This commercial illustrates the mentality of engaging in unhealthy behaviors and choosing to take a pill to offset the impact.

One of my patients, Dan, was a man in his thirties whose previous doctor put him on a statin medication to lower his cholesterol.

After reviewing Dan's history, it was clear that he did not necessarily need a statin medication, and instead, he needed to make therapeutic lifestyle changes.

When asked what advice this doctor had given him about diet, Dan said that the doctor said, "Don't worry too much about your diet; just take this pill, try not to eat too much cheese or meat, and you'll be fine." Well, he stopped the medication and began to make lifestyle changes aligned with the core DRESS Code elements. Within just two months, not only were his cholesterol levels lower, but his chronic knee pain was no longer there.

This is one of many examples demonstrating that how we live is more important than what medication or diagnosis we have. That's why the elements of the DRESS Code are critical in addressing the diseases of our time.

Another of my patients was a thirty-four-year-old vegan named Sonia. She did everything right in terms of diet, but she continued to suffer from gas, bloating, and persistent weight problems. After further consultation, I determined that Sonia had an irregular sleep pattern from a stressful work situation. This contributed to a lack of physical activity and social isolation. While this patient's diet was excellent, there was inadequate time spent on cultivating healthy relationships, exercising, managing stress, and getting adequate sleep.

After considering these elements, Sonia was able to resolve the conflicts at work by quitting her job (long overdue, according to her) and finding a better position. She began regularly going out with her friends and even found a couple of exercise buddies. Once the DRESS Code pieces aligned, the gas, bloating, and sleep issues resolved.

Marta, a successful business owner, had neglected her health for far too long. When I first met with her, I discovered she had high blood pressure and high cholesterol. With a family history of heart attack (one killed her father at age fifty-six), Marta was motivated to make changes. Marta had been eating mostly processed foods with high amounts of bad fats and sugar. She was stressed at work and did not have time for any physical activity.

After our initial consultation together, she began introducing healthier foods and monitored her blood pressure. We gradually shifted her diet over the course of weeks to a mostly whole food, plant-based diet. On the relationships front, Marta was happily married and had a strong relationship with her husband and children, so, I simply reinforced the importance of this as part of her care and engaged her husband to help with supporting Marta with her lifestyle changes.

Marta was mostly focused on work and consequently lived a rather sedentary lifestyle and was overweight. Whenever she would start an exercise program, she would find it challenging due to joint pain from the excess weight, which led to her not following through with it. I started her with just walking for about twenty minutes every day to begin with. The timing of the walk was set to break up her day between work and dinner.

Work stress was always a key factor for Marta, even though she was quite successful. We came up with a plan to address this by creating protected time for reflection, breathing exercises, and meditative walking. This, along with planning frequent small trips with her husband and children, worked well to improve her stress.

Finally, we looked at sleep. Marta suffered from sleep apnea, which interfered with her quality of sleep, and she began a program to treat this. Within four months, Marta lost twenty-five pounds, and her blood pressure began to normalize. Fast-forward another six months: Marta had lost a total of sixty-five pounds and was now off all medications for blood pressure. Her joint pain also improved with less weight and her anti-inflammatory diet and practices. This is a good example of how using all the DRESS Code elements can transform our life, even in a person who has let things go for a long time.

CHAPTER 10

DO-IT-YOURSELF (DIY) DRESS CODE LONGEVITY HACKS

A ll the DRESS Code elements are interconnected; there is a considerable overlap between them, and that is really by design. The elements reinforce one another and work together to help us achieve optimal health. When we ignore one, it is to the peril of the other elements and to our overall health. The purpose of the DRESS Code is to simply understand the core elements that need to be addressed for health and longevity to occur. If we can do our part with each of these elements as individuals and as a society, it will be easier for communities to optimize their DRESS Code and for us to maximize our potential for living long and healthy lives.

THE TOP DIY DRESS CODE LONGEVITY HACKS

To get you started on your optimal health journey, I have compiled some of the best science and experiences from around the world to provide you with specific recommendations. I have broken this down by each of the key DRESS Code elements. As always, ask your doctor before trying any of these or any other practices. You can try one, two, or three or more from each list and see how you feel. Read about it, ask your doctor, and connect with me on social media. I would love to hear how the elements of the DRESS Code have positively impacted your life.

Diet

What we eat is probably the single-biggest contributor to longevity. The data clearly shows that dietary factors are the number one risk for premature, preventable death, so if you get this right, you are well ahead of the curve in terms of your healthspan.

- Eat the rainbow—and I don't mean Skittles! Every plant-based food in nature has a special nutrient and delicious flavor along with it. Eating the rainbow means you will get many of the vitamins, minerals, and antioxidants you need to reduce oxidative stress, lengthen your telomeres, slow down aging, and feel amazing.

- Avoid Frankenfoods! These accelerate aging by acting as a negative epigenetic input to speed up aging at the cellular level with chronic inflammation, oxidative stress, and DNA damage. These ultra-processed foods also disrupt metabolism, shorten telomere length, and block the body's longevity pathways. These include diets high in fast food, red meat, processed meat, and sugar-sweetened beverages. The opposite is true for diets rich in whole fruits, vegetables, and real food.

- Eat fat—that's right, you heard me right. To clarify, eat good fat. Fat is an essential part of your diet. Good fats are found in nuts, seeds, avocados, extra-virgin olive oil, and in wild seafood like salmon, mackerel, and sardines. Saturated fat can be both good and bad; it can raise your good HDL cholesterol or raise your bad LDL cholesterol. With saturated fat, choose plant sources like coconut oil, which is also rich in plant antioxidants, or if you do eat limited dairy, choose butter or plain yogurt from grass-fed cows.

- Limit animal-based protein; choose plant sources like nuts, seeds, beans, and legumes instead. You don't need as much protein as you think. Most Americans eat too much protein, and this can lead to premature disease and aging. Choosing unprocessed plant sources is your best bet.

- Eat beans every day, as these can add up to four years to your life.

- Avoid EXCESS sugar. Excess sugar without fiber, a key part of the SAD, wreaks havoc on your systems and leads to metabolic syndrome, a common pathway to diabetes, heart disease, and obesity. Choose complex carbohydrates in real foods for good sources of sugar with fiber.

- *Hara Hachi bu!* Translation: Eat until you are 80 percent full! This Okinawan philosophy is part of their secret to longevity. One way to do this successfully is to follow the "twenty-minute rule." After you take your first bite of food, it can take up to twenty minutes for your brain to register satiety or fullness. Eat slower, more mindfully, and enjoy every morsel, then check in at twenty minutes. If you are no longer hungry, chances are you have had enough.

- Less is more. Eating less has direct links to longer lifespans in both animals and humans. Based on the research to date, caloric restriction engages multiple longevity pathways and could extend human life by as much as fifty years. Whether you restrict your portion size or simply engage in a form of intermittent fasting, with eating, less is more.

- Do not eat late at night. Finish eating by 8 p.m. at the latest; 7 p.m. is even better. Nighttime calories contribute more to weight gain and insulin resistance than daytime calories. Instead of snacking at night, consider drinking calming teas like chamomile, mint, or lemon balm.

- Drink water, then drink some more. Multiple studies have identified the link between optimal water intake of five or more glasses per day with decreased risk of heart attacks and longevity. Aim for 0.5 to 1 ounce per pound of body weight, so if you weigh 175 pounds, you should have at least eleven cups of water (8 ounces each) per day. If you are more active, you may need to drink more. If you drink coffee or alcohol, add three cups of water to make up for the water lost by one cup of these dehydrating beverages.

- Nothing is better than a home-cooked meal! According to one study, eating out twice a day was associated with a 95 percent increased risk of early death from cancer or heart disease! Obviously, not all restaurant food is bad, and, in fact, some venues are creating meals that are both delicious and nutritious. Still, getting into the habit of cooking is your best bet for physical (and financial) wellness. When cooking, use real food ingredients and avoid prepacked foods with ingredients you cannot pronounce or do not understand.

- Eat these superfoods every day: beans, cruciferous vegetables, berries, dark leafy greens, tree nuts (walnuts, pecans, pistachios, almonds), seeds (pumpkin, sunflower, chia, flax), extra-virgin olive oil, whole grains, and tea.

- Eat mostly plants. You can't go wrong if you eat mostly plants the way the healthiest centenarians in the Blue Zones do.

- Eat less meat. Long-lived people with great healthspans do not always consume meat, but when they do, they eat two ounces no more than five times a month. If you do eat meat, avoid processed meat; choose pasture-raised or grass-fed. The fact that organic, grass-fed meat is more expensive helps limit it to a treat, rather than a staple of every meal.

- Fish is the best meat! Research also showed that pesco-vegetarians, or pescatarians, live the longest, with lower risks for dementia and cardiovascular disease, likely due to the plant forward diet plus the healthy fats and minerals found in wild seafood.

- Eat more calories earlier, and don't eat anything after 8 p.m. Eating later can lead to diabetes, heart disease, obesity, and poor sleep, while eating earlier can have the opposite effect. Eating during the day makes more sense since we are more active and can burn off the calories as well. Nighttime is really the best time for our bodies to focus on restoration and metabolic housecleaning, not digestion. Simply changing the timing of our meals can have a huge impact on health and longevity.

- Try the Mediterranean Diet. Among all the diets out there, the Mediterranean Diet is the most researched diet. It is mostly plant-based, with wild seafood and very small, if any, amounts of meat. Check out oldwayspt.org, a great nonprofit organization that shows how to adapt this dietary pattern to different global traditional diets from around the world. The benefits of this dietary pattern are numerous, and include preventing heart attacks and strokes, improving depression and boosting mood, reducing chronic pain, preventing dementia, and increasing longevity.

- Stick to your diet plan for at least twenty-eight days before giving up. It takes twenty-eight days for your taste buds to reset and change your palate to crave healthier foods. When you go back to eating a processed Frankenfood after that, you will taste the overwhelming salt or sugar difference as compared to the real food you've grown used to. The best part is that your genes will literally change, and your inflammation and oxidative stress will decrease almost immediately after changing your diet.

Relationships

Our connections with one another and the quality of those relationships matter. Connecting with one another with a sense of meaning and purpose enhances longevity and well-being. Connections with nature, including animals, are part of this important DRESS Code element.

- Make time for love in your life. Social connections are one of the most important factors in a long and healthy life. Invest in authentic relationships. Loneliness kills, while connectedness gives us life. Having these relationships in life powerfully impacts our physical and mental health. Be social, and schedule this into your calendar, so you are not sitting at home on your smartphone or watching TV alone.

- Hug and kiss your loved ones every day. Hugging for at least thirty seconds every day releases oxytocin, which has all sorts of benefits to your mood, happiness, and overall health.

- Develop a circle of close friendships. If you are a man, make sure to have close friends, as men do poorer than women later in life because of the lack of social connectedness. This is especially true for widowers.

- Join a team. Being a part of teams for sports or games is a great strategy to stay connected with others. With sports, we combine the two DRESS Code elements of exercise and relationships. Leisure-time sports that involve more social interaction versus solo exercise routines are associated with longevity, adding as much as five years to your life.

- Engage with your faith community. Stay engaged with your fellow believers and live longer. Studies have shown that people active in their church or religious community are healthier and live longer.

- Connect with nature. In Japan, *shinrin-yoku* ("forest bathing") involves taking in all of nature. Spending time outdoors improves mental health, and even a single instance of forest bathing can reduce depression and anxiety symptoms, while providing renewed energy and feelings of calmness.

- Learn to forgive and let go of grudges. Carrying around the pain of someone who has wronged you is bad for your mental and physical health. Read about forgiveness with books like *Learning to Forgive* by Dr. Fred Luskin, and find out how this can improve your health, while making you feel happier in the process.

- Find your best furry friend. People with pets tend to have lower instances of depression and fewer health problems. In particular, dog owners have been found to live longer.

- Be truthful. Truthfulness is foundational to all virtues. Lying can undermine healthy relationships and contribute to poorer social connections. Being truthful with yourself and others is not only the ethical thing to do, but it can also help you stay connected to stay healthy.

- Serve others. When in doubt or troubled, try serving others. Research has shown that people who volunteer just five hours a month are happier than those who don't. Volunteers also have better ways of managing stress and a better sense of meaning and purpose in life.

- Limit social media use. Excessive use of social media contributes to loneliness, while using tools like virtual videoconferencing for real conversations with friends has the opposite effect. Invest in real friends, not toxic social media contacts.

- Find your partner in life. Consider getting married or committing to a long-term, monogamous, authentic, meaningful relationship. Married people who have quality relationships live longer for many reasons, including the social support and motivation to take care of themselves and each other in the process.

- Spend time with the kids. Engage with children and surround yourself with younger people to mentor, guide, and connect with. Studies show that people with children and older people who spend time with younger people live longer, so find ways to stay in touch with the younger crowd.

- Delay retirement—keep doing work you enjoy. Work is a great purpose for living. People who delay their retirement tend to live longer, and early retirement can be a risk factor for premature death.

- Be kind and generous; volunteer and serve others. Doing this will not only enhance your life, but will lengthen it as you connect with others and develop meaningful relationships.

Exercise

Of all the therapies that exist in the world, exercise is truly remarkable, as it impacts every part of our bodies and minds with more benefits than are listed here. When in doubt, just move!

- So, don't just sit there—move! Excessive sitting is dangerous! As Americans are now sitting for an average of seven hours a day, there is strong evidence to support the negative impact of excessive sitting on health and longevity. Even exercising for at least eleven minutes a day can make a huge impact on your risk of dying early. Don't sit for more than thirty minutes at a time, and when you get up from your chair, try doing ten squats and walk around the room for about five to seven minutes.

- Walk it out. Move naturally throughout the day. Walking at least a thousand steps a day can decrease your risk of dying of any cause by 28 percent. That's not to say you shouldn't exercise more, but even just walking a little bit every day can make a huge impact. Walking briskly at a pace of a hundred steps per minute after the age of forty is associated with even greater health and longevity. A recent study showed that just walking briskly for forty minutes three times a week in adults over the age of sixty increased white matter in the brain and improved memory. Start the habit today; almost everyone has time for a walk every day.

- Stay strong and stay healthy. Build and maintain muscle for as long as possible—muscle loss equals premature aging. People with more muscle strength at any age are less likely to die than people with less muscle mass. Muscle mass decreases with age. Without regular strength training, we will lose nearly 25 percent or more of our strength by age seventy. Strength training doesn't have to be intense; it can be just fifteen minutes a day. Ways to build strength through exercise include free weights, kettlebells, resistance bands, and using your own body weight.

- Sex is exercise. When we are intimate with our partners, we deepen our bonds together, which enhances the impact of relationships for health. Studies have shown that having regular sexual activity with your partner can reduce stress, inflammation, boost mood, and lower blood pressure. In one study of men in their forties and fifties, it even showed a decreased risk of dying by 50 percent!

- Consider high-intensity interval training (HIIT). This consists of short spurts of physical activity, alternating with intervals of rest or low-intensity activity. For example, on a treadmill, you can do two minutes at high speed or high elevation, followed by two minutes at low speed with a flat surface; alternate for twenty to thirty minutes (or you can just do this while walking on a path). HIIT literally reverses the age of your heart and your entire cardiovascular system.

- Sink or swim! Swimming is one of the best exercises. It's a total-body workout that is low impact, meaning you can do it with low risk of injury.

- Run for your life! Running is a key lifestyle medicine for longevity. Runners live longer, and almost any amount of running is beneficial, reducing your risk of premature death by as much as 30 percent.

Stress

Short-term stress can help us focus, and in the case of heat or cold therapy, it can reduce inflammation and heal us. Long-term stress in all its forms, whether arising from trauma or persistent sources, is toxic. Learning how to cope with it, change your perception of it, and reduce its impact are key parts of the longevity equation.

- Use a sauna or cold plunge or alternate between the two. Start with five minutes, hydrate, and try to increase after that (ask your doctor first). One way to try this on a less intense level is to just change the water temperature during your shower from warm to cool, then hot to cold each for a couple minutes. Again, discuss this with your doctor before trying this.

- Take a technology break. Take time every day away from electronics to reflect. Engaging in a reflective exercise like journaling reduces stress, boosts mood, and results in better coping skills in times of crisis. Even with your busy calendar, schedule time to reflect and de-stress.

- Try meditating. Meditation is one of the most powerful and time-honored tools to elicit the relaxation response, the state that reduces stress and inflammation. There are many forms of meditation to consider, from simple mantras to mindfulness. Whatever you choose, make sure you do it every day;

even just a few minutes a day can have a huge impact on your health and longevity.

- When in doubt, go for a walk or some other form of exercise. Exercise is a stress reliever and has a synergistic effect as another core DRESS Code element. Exercise enhances both physical and mental health. Whatever you decide to do is better than nothing, so don't sweat it as long as you just move!

- Engage in daily routines. Life is about rhythms, and this is important not only when it comes to sleep, but also for reducing the impact of stress and inflammation in your life. Following a routine allows your body to prepare for the next phase of your day, without having to stressfully react to an erratic schedule. The more consistent you are, the less chronic stress and inflammation you have.

- Whether you are young or old, try tai chi. This form of mind-body exercise has been around for literally thousands of years and has numerous health benefits. Based on exceptional evidence, the CDC recommends tai chi as the best treatment for fall prevention in the elderly.

- If you haven't tried yoga yet, you might want to consider it. Yoga is another mind-body therapy with numerous health benefits, including reducing stress and inflammation, and boosting strength.

- Mental health is as important as physical health. I'll say it again: Mental health is as important as physical health. If you have been diagnosed with depression or anxiety, get help. Untreated mental health problems result in chronic stress and inflammation that accelerate the aging process. Use all the tools you need to get better. You may not need medication and will definitely benefit from counseling and therapy to process things and shift your perspective for the better.

- Think positive—mindset is everything. If you perceive your health to be excellent, you have a higher likelihood of achieving a greater healthspan. Shifting your perspective is often the easiest and most profound thing you can do to cope with stress and reframe your reality. Shifting your perception enables you to achieve resilience and grit in life, a key factor in reducing stress and achieving your goals, no matter what life may bring.

- Find a sense of purpose and meaning in your life. Read the book *Man's Search for Meaning* by Viktor Frankl, and discover how finding meaning even in the direst circumstances can enable you to overcome the greatest challenges of life. Having meaning and purpose is a great way to reduce stress by having a defined path and striving toward it. You can find great joy in living your purpose every day.

- Don't stay in a stressful job or toxic relationship. Don't give up easily, instead, work on fixing it, and then decide what you can and can't do. Unhealthy relationships and stressful jobs can literally take years off your life.

- Just breathe. Sometimes the best thing you can do to relieve stress is to take a few quiet minutes every day to quiet your mind and focus on your breath. Start simply by sitting quietly for a few minutes without any devices or distractions, and pay attention to your breathing. Practice slower and deeper breathing, and try a meditative practice to elicit the relaxation response.

- Stay connected with nature. Connecting with nature is calming and reduces numerous inflammatory markers in your body. Depending on where you live, this may be as easy as just stepping outside for a few minutes every day.

- Take time off. As the saying goes, "Don't live to work; work to live." While working is important and provides a sense of purpose in life, it's possible for it to be too much of a good thing. This is especially true if our overworking results in less time to invest in your important relationships and taking care of yourself. Plan for vacations and take that time off to renew, de-stress, and recalibrate.

- Eat more fiber, which means eat more plants. Fiber from whole plant foods not only can decrease your risk of diabetes, heart disease, and cancers of the gastrointestinal track, but it can also boost your mood. A recent study suggests that eating more than 18.7 grams of fiber per day is linked to the lowest risk of moderate to severe depression.

- Practice gratitude. Reflect on what you are grateful for each day. Writing down the five things you are most grateful for every night boosts mood, increases optimism, and reduces stress levels. Gratitude is contagious, and your happiness will spread to your family and friends.

- Be playful and live like you are Peter Pan. Playing in whatever form is key to mental health and well-being. Learn not to take everything so seriously by taking time to play every day. This could be a game like tennis or just spending time playing with your kids; either way, play is a great way to reduce stress and stay healthy.

- Attitude is everything. Recognize that you can choose how you act in the face of life's challenges. Practice seeing the glass as half full, and you will benefit by seeing the silver lining in difficult situations.

- Recognize that you have the power of choice. You can always choose what to focus on, what things mean to you, and what to do despite any challenges or fears you have to overcome.

SLEEP

Sleep is the most underrated, underutilized tool to boost immunity, enhance healthspan, and help you feel better every day.

- Get your Zzzs! Most of us do not get enough sleep. While seven hours is associated with most of the benefits of sleep, closer to eight hours is ideal. After age sixty-five, getting between six and seven hours is probably fine.

- Practice good sleep hygiene. Dimming the lights two hours before bed, avoiding screen time forty-five minutes before bed, wearing protective blue light–blocking glasses to keep melatonin levels high, and avoiding excessive stimulation in your bedroom are all examples of sleep hygiene. Experiment for yourself and find a routine that fits with your life.

- Exercise every day and sleep well every night. Being physically active helps to improve the quality and quantity of your sleep. This is yet another example of how the DRESS Code elements complement one another.

- Have a regular nightly routine for sleep: Go to bed at the same time and wake up at the same time every day.

- Set your circadian clock with natural light. Exposing your eyes to natural light early in the morning and again in the late afternoon sets your internal clock to maximize melatonin levels for optimal sleep.

- Avoid stimulating activities at night. The more you try to be productive after dinner, the more difficult it will be for you to get quality sleep. This may seem like an impossible task, but one way to do this is by setting an alarm for stopping any work or stimulating activity. You can then get into the habit of stopping no matter what, so you can begin the process of slowing down and eventually falling asleep.

- Avoid caffeinated beverages after 4 p.m., and minimize alcohol as well. The later in the day we have these drinks, the worse our sleep will be. Focus on drinking water or a caffeine-free tea like chamomile as part of your sleep hygiene routine.

- Caffeine basically gives you a false sense of wakefulness, even though you are really depleted and need sleep. It's okay to drink coffee or tea, as there are health benefits to these beverages, but it is not okay to use these as a substitute for sleep.

- A chapter a day keeps the doctor away. Try reading a book at bedtime instead of scrolling through your phone. One study showed that people who read at least thirty minutes every day lived two years longer than non-readers. Reading also helps with falling asleep, lowers heart rate, eases muscle tension, and has a calming effect on your mind.

- If you want to nap, take a "power nap." A power nap of no more than thirty minutes (ideally about twenty minutes) can increase alertness and energy levels. Longer napping for greater than an hour every day has been linked to increased risk of death from any cause. A short nap, however, is a great way to recharge your batteries and relieve stress.

- Stop scrolling! These days, most of us bring our phones to bed, so it's important to remember that part of good sleep hygiene is avoiding screen time before bed. This is especially true for "doomscrolling"—excessively scrolling through social media feeds looking for negative updates. This only contributes to further stimulation and stress without any benefit. The same goes for arguing with strangers on social media platforms, which can often happen right before bed, resulting in increased stress and difficulty sleeping.

- Snoring and sleepy all day? If you experience daytime sleepiness and your partner tells you that you snore, consider doing a sleep study. Sleep apnea is more common than you think, and while being overweight or obese is a risk factor, it can occur in people with normal weight as well. Getting this diagnosed and treated can be a key part of getting a good night's sleep.

- No more all-nighters! This is disruptive to your sleep cycle, and while you might have been able to pull it off when you were younger, it's like withdrawing money from your sleep bank, without ever repaying yourself. It takes time and energy for your body to readjust the internal clock after staying up late—the same time and energy that could be used to knock out precancer cells and keep you healthy. So stick to your sleep schedule as much as possible.

CHAPTER 11

THE THIRTY-DAY DRESS CODE CHALLENGE

In just thirty days, you can literally change the expression of your genes and upgrade your software to become a better, healthier version of yourself. By making specific changes over thirty days in each of the DRESS Code elements, you will gain more energy and more clarity, and you will begin to reboot your system for an optimal health span.

Day One

On day one, take stock of where you have been and how far you have come. Recognize that you are on a path of change. This will not be easy, but it will change you for the better if you remember to stay focused and keep going. Sometimes it's two steps forward and one step back. As long as you press on, you will achieve your goals.

Many of us set ambitious goals for change and fail in the process. In fact, more than 80 percent of so-called New Year's resolutions fail by February. The reason for this has to do with a lack of specificity in goal setting and unrealistic expectations. When we take on too much too quickly, we can fail, and this is demoralizing. Another common pitfall is having too broad a goal or an all-or-nothing approach, which sets us up for failure.

Our brains are set up to be rewired and change our habits. We have only to tap into this process. What is required is quick success that reinforces a new behavior and builds momentum to make that change consistent over time. The best way to do this is by setting more specific, manageable, and achievable goals.

All we have to do is START by choosing one simple goal from each of the DRESS Code categories. START is an acronym for how to set a simple, achievable goal to get going and build the momentum you need to keep going. When looking at this goal, it is important for it to START well:

Specify It

Time It

Achieve It

Repeat It

Try Harder!

Your goal needs to be *specific*. Don't just plan to exercise more; in the next seven days, plan to walk three times a week or decide to eat a bowl of fresh berries every day. Go to sleep every night at the same time, and connect with friends at least twice in person, virtually, or on the phone. Download a meditation app and spend five minutes with it every day. Whatever goal you set in any of the DRESS Code elements, make sure it is specific.

Next, *time it*. Set a time for how long and when you will be undertaking your goal. If you plan to walk three days in the coming seven days, put it in your calendar with an exact time so this actually happens. If you plan to connect with two friends, decide who exactly and when to do this. Set the time now with them to make it happen. Schedule the time when you will eat those berries. You get the point—whatever you do, make sure to have it be time-bound and time-set.

Now comes the next most important part. *Achieve it!* You actually have to go through with it. When it comes time to do the specific activity, you have to do it! This is execution, and part of successful execution is making sure you've identified a specific time and task. The other part is making sure you haven't tried to take on too much too quickly.

Often, we try to be weekend warriors when it comes to exercise and end up overdoing it and injuring ourselves. Or we set too high a goal, such as going from being totally inactive to running every day for thirty minutes. Or maybe we decide to stop eating any dessert forever. These extreme goals are like New Year's resolutions that only last for the month of January and fade away soon after.

To achieve your goal, you need to make it something you can achieve. To achieve a goal, you should be able to rate it as seven or more on a ten-point scale of likelihood that you will achieve it. If you can't give it a seven or greater, you need to rethink your goal and try something a bit easier. Although you may think that a goal is just too easy, think again. Achieving a really easy goal is a key way to build momentum toward success. Better to start low and go up slowly than to aim too high, only to fall down too quickly before you've had a chance to get going.

Once you achieve it, it is important to celebrate that win, however small it is. This celebration reinforces the new behavior in our brain with a dopamine hit that is a healthy addiction. Now we can go on to the next step: repeating what we did and keep it going.

Once you have a specific, time-bound, time-set goal that is achievable, and you actually begin doing it, keep up the great work. Can you *repeat it*? Can you keep things going and do it again, or was this something you just did for a few days and let go of after that? You may want to keep the same goal for another week to make it stick. Once you feel you have it down, you can start adding more. Again, keep in mind that you don't have to rush it, but you don't want to just stay where you are.

Once you achieve your goal and repeat it, you can then begin to *try harder*! Add another fifteen minutes a week of walking or extend it to thirty minutes. You choose the next step. You have the power, and you control the pace. As long as you don't stagnate and get stuck in a rut, you can go up steadily and move forward when you feel ready. This is where listening to your body and allowing it to adjust to changes you have made become critical to achieving success. This is where you begin to build on your success and take it to the next level. You had the berries, now you add a bowl of fresh leafy greens and homemade salad dressing. Both of these are great initial steps to improving your diet.

You can pick a goal from one of the DIY List of Health Span Hacks in Chapter 10 that I have included as a way for you to get started on your path. Instead of prescribing a specific series of steps, I want to empower you to choose your own adventure. You can decide among these hacks or one of your own. You either will succeed or, if it's not optimal, you will learn and improve things from there.

The goals you choose are your own. The DRESS Code gives you the tools you need to make your own plan. This is the ultimate DIY approach. It's not something we can set for you, but we can share the process and tips on getting started. By not simply telling you what to do, you will be empowered with the tools you need to create a personalized plan for success. To help with this, I have put together a short workbook format below to help you get started.

Just START with Your DRESS Code Goals

Diet Goal

Relationships Goal

Exercise Goal

Stress Goal

Sleep Goal

Here are some examples of what you can choose and how it works. Follow the steps above to set a goal and then you can START. Make sure to pick at least one goal from each DRESS Code element.

Diet—Let's say you want to the following DIY Health Span Hack: Avoid excess sugar in all its forms. Let's say you eat processed foods and prepacked foods that contain sugar. You can set a goal to avoid added sugars in food products, and instead, focus on getting sugar as part of whole foods like fruits.

A great way to avoid excess sugar, as noted in the Diet chapter, is by reading labels to identify products that have "added sugars."

If you eat fast food more than three times a week, start by limiting it to one or two times a week. Or if you take on the sugar goal, start by reading labels and avoiding added sugars for at least half of your meals this week.

Relationships—Let's say you decide to invest in meaningful friendships by following the example of long-lived centenarians who enjoy regular outings every week with their group of close friends. Nowadays, this doesn't have to be in person; even setting up a virtual call with friends who may live far away will help fill this need.

Days 2–7

These are the days that you move forward with the goals you set on Day 1 for each of the DRESS Code elements.

Days 8–14

It's time to keep going! You may have achieved some of your goals for the first seven days and now the question is can you repeat it? With other goals, you may have fallen short, and that's okay. As Theodore Roosevelt famously said, "Man's greatest honor is not in never falling, but in rising every time we fall." And that's true with this thirty-day challenge and any path of change you set yourself on in life. There will ALWAYS be setbacks and even failures. But, as long as you keep getting back up and keep going, you will arrive at a better place than where you are today.

This is the time to keep going with the goals you have achieved—it's time to achieve them again and make the habit stick. Can you keep the new momentum going and build on it? I believe you can, because you have decided the goals and are now achieving them in all the DRESS Code elements. Even one goal with each element can have a huge impact on your sense of well-being.

Days 15–21

By now, you have begun to establish some nice routines, and you may want to consider the next step of getting a good START. Namely, you can START to try harder! This may not be the case for every goal you have set, but for some of them, you may be ready to try a bit harder.

When adding more to a goal, keep the same formula in mind as when you STARTed. Make sure it is something you can Specify, Time, Achieve, and Repeat before making it your next step. Remember that doing too much too quickly can set you back, but pushing yourself at the right time will give you the edge you need to take things to the next level.

As Socrates is thought to have said, "Know thyself." Knowledge is power, and knowing who you are allows you to be honest with where you are. This will allow you to set realistic goals and gradually increase them to the next stage of difficulty. Having a partner or close friend to help you along the way can be an important part of this. If you are married or have a partner, make sure they know you are taking the Thirty-Day DRESS Code Challenge. Even better would be for you to both do the challenge together. While your goals may be different, doing it together will only reinforce your ability to stay accountable and keep moving forward.

Days 21–28

By this week, you are starting to realize that your software is being upgraded all over your body! The DRESS Code has been unlocked and is beginning to work its magic. Key physiological changes happen throughout your body and in your brain to recalibrate to a healthier you. Telomere length is stabilizing; aging processes are slowing and optimizing. You will likely feel more energy and experience better moods than when you started. You will get more restful sleep and cultivate important relationships in your life. You can begin to see the light at the end of the tunnel, and things are finally starting to look better than they have in a long time.

Your taste buds have been reset! That's right. All it takes to reset your taste buds is twenty-eight days, and you made it. If you want to prove it to yourself, try to eat a candy bar or other sugary processed food that you used to eat. You won't need to take more than a few bites before feeling overwhelmed by the taste of pure sugar. If your goal was to cut out added salt and high-sodium foods (the same processed foods high in sugar are also high in sodium), then you will taste pure salt. This will reinforce the fact that you are no longer desensitized to this overload of salt or sugar in your diet.

Days 29 and 30

You made it! Celebrate how far you have come. Reflect on what happened, where you are now, and where you were when you began. How is your *diet* now? How are your *relationships*? Do you move your body and *exercise* more regularly? How is your level of *stress*? How much good quality *sleep* do you get every night?

Take the time to celebrate your wins and reflect on your losses. Decide what's next. Where you go from here is up to you. I recommend you continue to establish your new habits and upgrade your software, changing your genes for the better. There's no reason to stop—the cycle can continue, and the next level of goals and achievements will come your way.

CHAPTER 12

HOW TO NAVIGATE OUR SICK CARE SYSTEM AND USE THE DRESS CODE TO OPTIMIZE YOUR HEALTH

As discussed earlier, we do not have a "health" care system—rather, we have a reactive, disease-management, "sick" care system. While treating disease and acutely life-threatening conditions is critically important, preventing these from happening is a more proactive and impactful approach. Remember the DRESS Code curve: shifting to the right to increase our healthspan.

The DRESS Code enables us to hone in on the key biohacking elements that can help us live healthier for longer. But the question is how to navigate our current "sick" care system to get the data and care that we need to effectively be proactive about our health?

Knowing Is Half the Battle

Knowledge is power, and knowing is half the battle. Knowing your numbers and recognizing your risk factors are critical! Without this knowledge, you cannot begin to address what is there and take the key steps to unlocking your greatest health and longevity. When it comes to our health, there are now a variety of ways to learn more about where we stand in terms of our biological age and health status.

Getting that annual physical or screening test for precancer or early-stage disease can literally make the difference between life and death. Screening tools have long been used successfully to save lives. Additionally, knowing where we stand can make a big difference for motivation and a sense of urgency regarding next steps. Colonoscopies are a great example of this, as finding early-stage precancerous polyps can make the difference between a simple removal and a fatal cancer diagnosis.

Thankfully, there are now even more ways to detect disease in early stages. With these new technologies, we can detect cancer much earlier than ever before and find a heart attack brewing years before it happens. In the book *Life Force*, Tony Robbins and Drs. Peter Diamandis and Robert Hariri share some of these newer screening tools and breakthrough therapies. It is an exciting time, as with some of these emerging technologies, we are beginning to find innovative and effective ways to find disease before it takes root and prevent it from causing us harm. We are also finding new ways to treat old conditions. While some of this is accessible now, much of it is still being researched and disseminated.

But even more important than what is discovered through early-stage screening is what we can do about it now. For example, advanced MRI imaging and computer algorithm technologies can identify visceral fat levels and detect potential for conditions like heart disease or diabetes. When combining these tests with an assessment of the DRESS Code elements in our lives, we can create powerful tools to proactively detect early-stage disease and discover actionable insights to prevent illness, optimize our health, and expand our healthspan for longer than ever before.

Key Labs and Tests

Most of us would benefit from an annual physical exam. Most doctors will perform an exam and the following lab tests:

- Complete metabolic panel (This test measures metabolism, including kidney and liver function markers, as well as electrolytes and blood sugar for the day of the test.)

- Complete blood cell count with differential (This includes a complete cell count of all cell types to check for anemia and blood disorders.)

- Thyroid stimulating hormone with reflex for T4 (This checks our thyroid function with initial screening tests.)

- Lipid panel (This is the test for our cholesterol and needs to be done fasting for at least ten hours prior for most accurate results.)

In addition to the above, I also recommend the following tests at least annually, and possibly more often, depending on the results:

- Hemoglobin A1c (This test screens for diabetes and includes a three-month average of blood sugar control.)

- Vitamin D level (Vitamin D is now considered more of a hormone-like thyroid with a far-reaching impact on almost every system in our body.)

- Vitamin B12 (This is connected with energy levels, the ability of our cells to repair DNA, and links to our brain function and cognitive skills.)

- TSH + T4 + T3 and optionally thyroglobulin antibodies and thyroid peroxidase antibody tests (This gives a fuller picture of your thyroid function and also screens for autoimmune destruction of your thyroid.)

- Uric Acid (This tests for markers for gout and inflammation.)

- Homocysteine (This test measures an amino acid that increases oxidative stress, inflammation, and insulin resistance, which is an independent marker for heart disease and B12 metabolism; if levels are high, you can consider a regimen of methylated B vitamins.)

- A coronary CT calcium score (This test measures a marker for coronary artery disease; a score of zero is reassuring, while a score of 200 can indicate the need for further testing to rule out narrowing of your coronary arteries.)

- Additional tests to consider:

   o Micronutrient testing to see where your body is in terms of many micronutrients like zinc, selenium, magnesium, and others. Eating the rainbow of mostly whole plant foods with nuts and seeds will give you many of these key nutrients, but many of us may still not be getting adequate amounts. This test can give us a picture of where we are and what dietary changes and potential supplements are needed.

What Do My Cholesterol Numbers Mean?

The standard lipid panel gives us several values, including total cholesterol, high-density lipoprotein (HDL), calculated low-density lipoprotein (LDL), and triglycerides. It will also calculate very low-density lipoprotein (VLDL).

While risks vary for each person depending on other factors, such as smoking status, weight, blood pressure, or age, it is important to recognize some general concepts when it comes to cholesterol.

LDL cholesterol and VLDL (the percentage of LDL that is lower density) is known as "bad" cholesterol. This is the cholesterol most susceptible to damage that leads to inflammation and narrowing of our arteries over time, which increases our risk for a heart attack or stroke. The theory behind lowering LDL is that the less LDL we have, the lower our risk for it to get damaged and eventually lead to heart disease. That's why statin medications were developed and hailed as a huge success. Statin medications lower LDL and have little to no effect on HDL, total cholesterol, or triglycerides.

Outside of a small percentage of people with genetically high LDL from cholesterol disorders, for most of us, LDL comes from animal protein and fat in our diet. If you eat a whole food, plant-based diet, your LDL will decrease dramatically, similar to the effect of taking a statin medication.

It is better to lower LDL with diet and lifestyle changes, rather than taking a statin. Statins, like most medications, do not come without side effects. Statin side effects include liver damage; thinking or memory difficulties that results in instances of confusion, sexual dysfunction, and fatigue; and muscle aches and pains.

Most statins, except for pravastatin, will also increase your risk for insulin resistance and diabetes. If your LDL and other risk factors are not too high (e.g. > 150) and you have no evidence for narrowing of arteries anywhere in your body, you are better off not taking a statin.

For people who have had a heart attack, stroke, or known heart disease anywhere in the body, the research supports taking a statin to prevent further life-threatening events. However, even in these cases, it is best to optimize all the DRESS Code lifestyle elements and take the lowest effective statin dose to minimize the risk for side effects.

I always recommend taking a CoQ10 supplement (usually 100 to 200mg daily with food that contains fat) if you are going to take a statin medication. The reason is that CoQ10 is a co-enzyme in our mitochondria (the energy building units of our cells) that gets depleted when we take statin medications. This supplement helps to offset some of the mentioned potential side effects of statin medications.

Additionally, even for people with heart disease or history of a heart attack or stroke who can benefit from a statin, making lifestyle changes is still necessary and hugely impactful. I will discuss how I approach this with patients in these cases by applying the DRESS Code later in this chapter.

About half of people who have heart attacks or strokes have normal or low LDL levels. This tells us that LDL is not the whole story. In fact, the Mediterranean Diet has a larger effect than statin drugs (reducing risk for another heart attack or stroke in those with a history by more than 70 percent, versus 35 percent decreased risk, as shown in the best statin medication research studies). While the Mediterranean Diet has little to no effect on LDL levels, it does impact both triglycerides and HDL levels. The triglyceride-to-HDL ratio is a key risk factor independent of LDL levels.

Triglycerides come from sugar or simple refined carbs and grains in our diet. This can include sugary beverages, as well as alcoholic beverages. Simple carbs are a big part of the SAD as discussed earlier. So it is not surprising to find many of us with higher-than-normal triglyceride levels. By decreasing our intake of sugary beverages and simple carbs by eating whole food sources of fiber with complex carbs (basically any plant food, not juice), we can decrease our triglycerides. Additionally, omega-3 fish oil supplements taken with food (around 3 to 5 grams of EPA + DHA daily) have been shown to decrease triglyceride levels by up to 50 percent.

HDL is known as the "good" cholesterol. Cardio/aerobic exercise can raise HDL. Healthy fats (nuts, seeds, extra-virgin olive oil), as well as saturated fat, also raise one's LDL. That's why saturated fat is a double-edged sword, in that it can raise both HDL and LDL levels.

The triglyceride/HDL is a marker for insulin resistance and an independent risk factor for heart attacks and strokes. A triglyceride/HDL of greater than 5 is associated with a much higher risk (up fourteen times more) for a heart attack or stroke, independent of the LDL level. A lower triglyceride/HDL ratio of less than 2 is associated with a much lower risk for heart attack and stroke. Therefore, in my practice, I focus on the triglyceride/HDL ratio and LDL when I look at cholesterol levels for my patients.

Ask Your Doctor about Lifestyle Changes

As many as two-thirds of doctors' visits in the United States result in a prescription medication. While medications can be lifesaving, adverse drug effects are ranked between the fourth and sixth leading cause of death in the United States.

We should not rely solely on medications for our care. Dr. Andrew Weil has written a great book, *Mind Over Meds*, that documents the tenfold increase in the use of both prescription and over-the-counter medications over the past fifty years. In his book, Dr. Weil discusses when medications are useful and when they are not. He also discusses how we can use diet and lifestyle or evidence-based supplements, which are safer than medications, to treat many common conditions, such as high blood pressure.

One of the key takeaways from his book is the idea that we should not take a medication for every symptom we have or a "pill for every ill," as the saying goes. When talking with your doctor, it is important to ask if there is an alternative to taking medication.

For example, with high blood pressure, depending on the cause and how high it is, you can ask your doctor if there is anything other than or in addition to medication that you can do. A good physician will tell you that your diet, physical activity level, and the other DRESS Code lifestyle elements will substantially impact your blood pressure. Using diet and lifestyle as a first-line approach is key to most health conditions.

Finding the Right Doctor

In an ideal world, everyone would have a primary care physician. In countries where there are enough primary care doctors for everyone, people live healthier for longer, with less hospitalizations and costs associated with their medical care. In the United States, where our "sick" care system does not value primary care by literally paying these critical doctors much less than other specialties, our health outcomes are much poorer and more expensive.

Despite spending more on healthcare than any other nation on earth, we have some of the worst health outcomes and lead the developed world in chronic disease. One key solution to this problem is to ensure that everyone has access to a primary care doctor who knows you and can develop a relationship with you over time to keep you healthy. So, if you do not have a primary care doctor now, it is important to find one you like and who enjoys working with you.

While all physicians, including all primary care doctors, are happy to see their patients make positive lifestyle changes, not all physicians are trained with the expertise to support you in optimizing your health with the DRESS Code.

For example, when it comes to diet, medical doctors only get an average of 19.6 hours of nutrition education across all four years of medical school. While it is important to seek care when acutely ill by going to your primary care doctor (if you are lucky enough to have one) or the urgent care or emergency room, finding the right doctor to help you make the changes you need to stay healthy is arguably even more important as we age.

Most of us would benefit from seeing a doctor certified in lifestyle medicine by the American College of Lifestyle Medicine. Lifestyle medicine training includes six pillars that parallel the core elements of the DRESS Code. These include nutrition, physical activity, stress management, restorative sleep, social connections, and avoiding risky substances that can cause harm through addiction (this includes drugs, alcohol, and tobacco products). Physicians who have had this training have the expertise to guide you on how to make the lifestyle changes you need to optimize your health.

Their focus is primarily on lifestyle changes to treat risk factors for disease like high blood pressure or high cholesterol, instead of relying on medications. These physicians will also prescribe intensive lifestyle changes to treat and even reverse chronic medical conditions, such as type 2 diabetes or heart disease.

One well-known example for reversing heart disease through lifestyle changes is the Ornish Program. This program, which includes all the DRESS Code lifestyle components, has been shown to reverse plaque formation in coronary arteries in a matter of months.

This is amazing, considering that many people with clogged arteries have to have stents implanted to keep them open. The Ornish Program accomplishes this with a whole-food, plant-based diet, stress reduction, exercise, social support, and meditation.

Research supports this and other examples of a lifestyle-medicine approach, and many patients have reversed their chronic disease by making the changes recommended by their lifestyle medicine physician. To learn more about these doctors and where to find one, visit the American College of Lifestyle Medicine.

Many of us can benefit from seeing an integrative medicine physician. According to Dr. Weil, integrative medicine is "a healing-oriented medicine that takes into account the whole person (body, mind, and spirit), including all aspects of lifestyle. It emphasizes the therapeutic relationship and uses of all appropriate therapies, both conventional and alternative."

Physicians who practice integrative medicine neither reject conventional medicine nor accept alternative therapies without evidence. These physicians usually complete a one- or two-year fellowship in integrative medicine, where they learn about different care modalities, such as TCM, Ayurvedic medicine, as well as the use of supplements and herbs as part of treatment protocols.

These physicians can dive deeper into the root causes of illness, and not simply treat symptoms, by taking a whole-person approach to care. A great resource for finding an integrative medicine physician is the online database of alumni of the Andrew Weil Center for Integrative Medicine.

While 80 to 90 percent of us will benefit from both a lifestyle medicine- and integrative medicine-trained physician for both primary and specialty care, some of us have more complicated conditions that may need even more extensive testing and evaluation. In these situations—such as long COVID, fibromyalgia, Lyme disease, or unexplainable symptoms that are not improved adequately by lifestyle changes—a bit more of a medical mystery needs to be solved.

In these cases, the Institute for Functional Medicine is a great resource for finding doctors who have expertise in this field. Sometimes, you can even find doctors certified in both integrative and functional medicine, who can help with a wider variety of complicated conditions.

What about Supplements?

Many patients ask me about supplements. Some doctors feel supplements are ineffective and tell their patients that all supplements are a waste of money, or even worse, dangerous. The truth is that not everyone needs supplements, but many people can benefit from dietary supplements to reinforce their healthy lifestyle changes. And often, herbal remedies in the form of dietary supplements are safer than medications.

One of the challenges with supplements in the United States is that they are not regulated like pharmaceutical drugs. This means there are a wide variety of quality-control issues with the supplements you can buy. Some supplements don't even contain what the label says they do or even have been found to include trace levels of unhealthy substances, such as lithium or lead. The key here is to find a doctor who is well versed in vetting supplement companies and getting a more nuanced recommendation on what brands of supplements and doses to take.

Those of us who have completed a fellowship in integrative medicine learn extensively about herbal medicine and dietary supplements. We learn about when they are useful, what brands are reputable, and how and when they can potentially interact with medications.

In my integrative medicine practice, I routinely review my patients' supplements and help them get rid of the ones that are a waste of money or potentially harmful. I also review potential herb-drug interactions with these supplements and the medications they are taking. I then recommend evidence-based supplements that can help them with their health goals. Often, these supplements or herbal medicines can help people avoid or reduce medication intake.

As many as 42 percent of Americans are vitamin D deficient, and this number rises to 62 percent of Hispanic adults, and nearly 82 percent of African Americans. Lower vitamin D levels are associated with increased risk for depression, cancer, heart disease, and diabetes, and are connected to increased risk for severe illness and death from a COVID-19 infection.

Most research has established an ideal range of vitamin D levels to be between 60 and 80ng/ml, even though the cutoff for "normal" for most labs is set as low as 30ng/ml. Vitamin D is a fat-soluble vitamin, so you can't simply take it without monitoring your levels, since taking too much can lead to accumulation and toxicity. I routinely screen my patients for vitamin D and supplement them with vitamin D3 to improve their health outcomes. Vitamin D should not be taken at night, as it can suppress melatonin levels, which can interfere with sleep.

Vitamin B12 is another supplement to consider. Vitamin B12 deficiency is directly linked to type 2 diabetes and can also impact homocysteine levels. Vitamin B12 is poorly absorbed by many of us, so I usually recommend a sublingual version that basically dissolves under your tongue.

This version of B12 is like a B12 shot, as it gets directly absorbed into your bloodstream. Unlike vitamin D, B12 is water soluble, so it does not accumulate, as you urinate out the excess. Therefore, getting higher readings—even above normal—in blood tests for B12 is ideal. I usually recommend methylated B12 for optimal absorption, as some of us with MTHFR mutations have difficulty absorbing non-methylated forms. B12 should not be taken later than 4 p.m., as it can help boost energy, and if taken at night, can interfere with sleep.

Magnesium is another supplement with far-reaching effects, including lowering the risk for type 2 diabetes. Many of us are low in magnesium because we do not eat enough nuts and seeds (pumpkin seeds are high in magnesium, for instance) in our diet.

Different forms of magnesium have different benefits. Magnesium glycinate helps with sleep and stress, magnesium citrate helps with constipation, magnesium malate can help with chronic fatigue and fibromyalgia, magnesium threonate can help with brain health and cognition, and magnesium taurate can help with blood pressure.

Turmeric comes from the Curcuma longa plant, which is mostly grown in India and Southeast Asia. Turmeric can be eaten as a spice in food, and is better absorbed with fat and black pepper. It is filled with curcuminoids, which are active phytochemicals that have many health benefits, including blocking many intracellular pathways to cancer formation.

Some of the other benefits of turmeric include reducing the risk of blood clots, reducing inflammation, reducing depression symptoms, boosting skin health, improving blood sugar levels, and helping with pain relief. Studies show that turmeric supplementation is the equivalent of ibuprofen for arthritis pain relief. Other research shows that turmeric may lower the risk of colon cancer by preventing the growth of colon polyps.

Turmeric is poorly absorbed, so if you use this for joint pain or inflammation, you should take it with fat or black pepper to aid with absorption.

Zinc is a key part of wound healing and immunity. A safe daily amount of 30mg is a good idea for most of us, and more can be used if we are sick or exposed to viruses during cold or flu season. You can also check your zinc level with a simple blood test to ensure you are not too low or high.

Extra-virgin olive oil (EVOO), although not a supplement, can be used as a supplement and as a superfood. This is the star of the Mediterranean Diet. Studies show that those who consumed the most calories from EVOO have the lowest risk for heart attacks, strokes, and all causes of death.

EVOO is packed with phytonutrients that are strongly anti-inflammatory, including oleocanthal, which has a strong antioxidant activity that helps neutralize oxidative stress associated with aging. These compounds in EVOO also stabilize LDL and protect it from being damaged. Three and a half tablespoons of EVOO are equivalent to about 225mg of ibuprofen in terms of an anti-inflammatory effect without the side effects. (Ibuprofen side effects include high blood pressure and gastritis, or bleeding in the gastrointestinal tract.)

There are, unfortunately, many fake olive oils out there. Here's how to tell a quality EVOO: Make sure it is extra-virgin and from a single origin, ideally organic, and in a dark glass bottle. When you take a teaspoon of real, high-quality EVOO, it should give you a biting aftertaste that catches in your throat with a burning sensation that makes you want to cough. This is an indicator of higher polyphenol levels (plant chemicals) that are bioactive in giving you the health benefits.

The key with EVOO and all oils is making sure it does not get to the smoking point during cooking, as when it does, it gets damaged and forms trans fats. The key is to cook with as little oil as possible on lower heat, and then add EVOO as a finishing oil on top of your food or eat it by the spoonful.

Another set of supplements to consider are those that can boost immunity to help prevent and shorten the duration of upper respiratory infections like colds and flus.

- Vitamin D

  As noted above, ensuring you are not deficient in vitamin D is protective for a variety of health conditions. During the height of the COVID-19 pandemic, those who were vitamin D deficient had a higher risk of more severe illness, hospitalization, and death from a COVID-19 infection. So, it is a good idea to optimize your levels.

- Quercetin

  Quercetin is found abundantly in apples and onions, which is probably one reason why eating these foods daily has been associated with lower risks of cancer, all causes of mortality, and improved immune function. Quercetin can be taken as a supplement and has a special ability to inhibit progression of viruses like COVID-19 by binding to its receptors and inhibiting it from replicating throughout the body. Quercetin is strongly anti-inflammatory and can also reduce inflammation related to things like asthma or arthritis. One precaution is that it has a blood-thinning effect (similar to omega-3 fish oil), so careful consideration must be made if you are on a blood thinner. As always, ask your doctor before starting any of these supplements.

- N-Acetylene-Cysteine (NAC)

  NAC is the supplement version of cysteine, an essential amino acid. NAC can replenish glutathione, which is an essential antioxidant system in our body. Glutathione scavenges free radicals and reduces inflammation from the wear and tear of life. Clinically, NAC is often used to prevent or treat acetaminophen toxicity as a protective detoxifying compound for both the liver and the kidneys. Studies have even shown NAC helping with mental health by regulating the brain's glutamate levels, its most important neurotransmitter. It is also helpful for lung conditions and lung health, as it reduces inflammation through glutathione pathways in the lungs.

For any virus, the above supplements can help with the addition of higher doses of zinc and vitamin D in the short term. Some herbs can help with the common cold or flu, but can worsen a COVID-19 infection. These include echinacea, elderberry syrup, and Umcka.

Probiotics are also helpful, as studies have shown that supplementing with these during cold and flu season results in fewer infections, shortened duration of symptoms, and fewer absences from school.

The key to probiotics is multiple strains, not just one or two, but ten to twelve, and about 30 billion colony forming units (CFUs), usually stored in the refrigerator. As we learn more about the microbiome, we find that eating a plant-based or plant-forward diet (80 percent whole plant foods) with fiber is critically important.

Additionally, instead of popping probiotic pills all year round, try regularly consuming fermented foods that will continually replenish the diversity of your good bacteria to keep you healthy. These can include sauerkraut (cultured), kim chi, miso, tempeh, kefir, or yogurt (without added sugar and other unnecessary ingredients).

A Word about Alcohol

As of the writing of this book, research has advanced in our understanding of the dangers of alcohol consumption. While tobacco is generally recognized as a major cause of cancer, alcohol is not. In fact, many of us have grown up in cultures and societies where alcohol is seen as necessary to have fun and enjoy life. This may be at weddings, where everyone raises a glass, or on a vacation, where the expectation is for us to drink to unwind.

Unfortunately, if our goal is to live a longer, healthier, happier life, drinking alcohol regularly is not the best choice. The latest data now show that the studies in the 1980s and 1990s that supported alcohol consumption (specifically red wine) were flawed. When researchers went back and controlled for the error of misclassifying former drinkers as "never drinkers," the J curve showing apparent benefit to moderate drinking disappeared.

This means there is no net benefit to drinking moderately, as was previously thought.[35] In fact, the data now strongly suggests that the dangers of alcohol outweigh the potential benefits, including for antioxidants in red wine. The fact is, you can get the same antioxidants that protect against heart disease and dementia from superfoods like organic blueberries, blackberries, red or black grapes, and pomegranates.

There is now growing scientific consensus that there is no safe amount of alcohol (there was a recent announcement in 2025 by the Surgeon General asking for a cancer warning on alcohol products similar to tobacco). In fact, alcohol is the third-leading preventable cause of cancer in the United States. It is linked to over 100,000 cancer cases and more than 20,000 deaths each year.

Globally, alcohol use is been ranked the seventh-leading risk factor for premature death and disability, resulting in three times the loss of healthy years than all illicit drugs combined. Even small amounts can disrupt our hormones, damage our DNA, and fuel cancer growth.

According to the American Cancer Society, women who consume more than one alcoholic drink per day have a 10 to 15 percent higher risk of breast cancer compared with non-drinkers. Alcohol itself is linked directly to at least seven different kinds of cancer.

Additionally, there are other health implications of alcohol use. A study in 2022 showed that even one drink of alcohol in a middle-aged person can destroy both gray and white matter in the brain, contributing to premature aging and brain degeneration. Another recent study showed that alcohol reduces muscle synthesis by 25 percent. This relates to premature aging in the form of sarcopenia, where we need to maintain muscle mass to live healthier for longer.

Additionally, while alcohol seems to have a calming effect initially, it actually raises your baseline stress levels over time, making it a negative epigenetic input for stress on our bodies. In addition to these well-established risks, alcohol impairs judgment and is related to numerous fatalities, such as motor vehicle accidents.

In my clinical practice, I can recall several patients who benefited greatly by stopping alcohol altogether. One patient, Jan, was a sixty-year-old woman who had struggled for more than twenty years with insomnia, which had worsened after menopause. She had committed to healthy lifestyle changes and had optimized all DRESS Code elements, but was still having trouble sleeping. Jan admitted to me that she would routinely have one to two glasses of red wine every night. I told her that while alcohol is a depressant, it actually interferes with several phases of sleep. I advised her to stop drinking for one month to see how that impacted her.

I saw Jan four weeks later in the clinic, and she was excited to tell me that after the first week, she experienced "the best sleep" of her life. Now she had even more energy every day, and her mood was better than ever, just by going dry.

Another patient, Joe, was a typical guy who drank lots of beer. He was otherwise healthy and tried to live an active lifestyle. One thing he could never get rid of as much as he worked out and ate healthy was his belly. He did everything right, except for the beer. His wife was also my patient, so the three of us talked through it.

After a few visits, he stopped drinking alcohol completely for two months. Remarkably, the belly that would never go away decreased in size and disappeared completely at the end of the eight weeks. And, like Jan, Joe also felt a surge of newfound energy that he thought was gone because he was past his prime. He had more clarity of thinking and better sleep, as well.

If you want to try going dry, be positive about it. It is not about guilt or what you should be doing; it's about deciding to make a change for your health and longevity. Going dry also does not mean isolating yourself socially from others. Many long-lived cultures engage in drinking as part of their social connections. As discussed, investing in these relationships are critically important for our health and wellbeing. So, whether you are looking to connect with friends at 5 for happy hour or enjoy life's milestones or take much needed time for rest and relaxation, enjoy the experience and know that while these activities are required for a healthier life, the alcohol that is usually involved is optional. Enjoying life while going dry is a simple, yet strong and impactful way to help you live healthier for longer. Remember, when it comes to alcohol, less is definitely more.

DRESS Code for Diabetes

I have spoken about Miguel's case, and I have had the privilege of working with many other people like him to help reverse type 2 diabetes. Here is the general approach I take for people with this condition.

Diet

With type 2 diabetes, diet plays a critical role. For most of us who eat the SAD, we have way too many calories coming from refined grains and simple carbs. So, one of the first components of my food prescription is to stop Frankenfoods and avoid simple carbs, including things like sugary beverages. I also recommend not using diet products; research has shown that diet soda can worsen our risk for diabetes even more than regular soda (likely because of how this disrupts our endocrine system).

As with other conditions, I recommend a whole, plant-based diet, plus healthy fats from mostly plant sources, including EVOO, nuts, and seeds, as well as some wild seafood, if desired. Another food that can be used as medicine for diabetes is vinegar. Any form of vinegar lowers blood sugar as much as medication for diabetes. I generally recommend at least two teaspoons or more with meals, which can easily be put together with your own homemade salad dressing when combining it with EVOO and spices like cayenne or black pepper and Himalayan pink salt.

A key part of ensuring success with the food prescription for diabetes is to monitor your blood sugar. Knowledge is power. By monitoring your blood sugar daily with a standard glucometer (checking fasting and two hours after lunch and dinner) or a continuous glucose monitor, you can make key connections between what you eat, your activity level, and your blood sugar. This instantly reinforces what you need to do to bring the numbers down, and engages you to treat this like a daily game. Great examples of biohacking are wearable technologies (such as a smartwatch or an Oura ring) to get real-time data that helps us make lifestyle changes to optimize health.

Relationships

For diabetes, as with any chronic condition, relationships are important to ensuring follow-through and engagement with making lifestyle changes. In the case of Miguel, I was able to do this by engaging his wife and family in the changes that were needed. Making sure to include spouses and other key individuals in the care plan ensures accountability and support.

Exercise

Exercise will lower blood sugar every time. Just moving from being inactive to walking every day can have a big impact on diabetes. In fact, a short five- to ten-minute walk after every meal actually lowers blood sugar like a medication. Physical activity is a great complement to the dietary changes involved in treating diabetes, as outlined above. Seeing the impact of activity on blood sugar by checking the numbers every day is an important part of this process.

Stress

Chronic negative stress increases blood sugar levels and worsens diabetes. Ensuring a stress management plan through activities like meditation or yoga, which can lower stress, is a key part of approaching this for people with diabetes. In addition, hot or cold therapy, like a sauna or cold plunge, can also help reverse insulin resistance. Managing stress will improve blood sugar, so this is another key to treating and reversing diabetes.

Sleep

Inadequate sleep has been linked to insulin resistance and diabetes. One reason for this is that the changing hormones that lead to craving unhealthy foods increase this risk. Ensuring adequate sleep will help improve blood sugar levels and reduce insulin resistance.

Each person is different when it comes to what components of the DRESS Code play a larger role, so looking at each of these will help you see what next steps to take.

DRESS Code for Heart Disease

Tom came to me after suffering his first heart attack at age sixty-one. His blood pressure was higher than normal, and his cholesterol reading was: TC 205 (slightly high), triglycerides 285 (high),

HDL 35 (low), LDL 136 (moderate), and VLDL 40 (high). Tom had thought he was healthy, although after discussing his diet and lifestyle, we discovered several areas that likely contributed to his risk for the heart attack.

Diet

Tom's diet was mostly "meat and potatoes," with fast food three to four times per week. We discussed the key role that diet plays in health, and I gave him a food prescription. I advised him to stop eating fast food and explained the difference between real food and Frankenfoods. I also helped him transition to a mostly whole-food, plant-based diet that is a variation of the Mediterranean Diet. This diet included plenty of whole fruits and vegetables, as well as raw nuts (especially tree nuts, including pecans, pistachios, almonds, and walnuts). I also included about six to eight tablespoons of EVOO with food per day.

Relationships

Tom was married with two adult children, so it was important for me to emphasize the importance of these relationships. Tom was admittedly stressed out from work, even though he was in a good financial position and did not need to work as much as he did. Tom didn't realize how important relationships were for his health, so we discussed cutting back on work and spending more time investing in his relationships with family and close friends.

Exercise

Tom had a mostly sedentary lifestyle. In the past, he had enjoyed tennis and hiking, but had not made time for this due to his work schedule. In cutting back from work and connecting more with family and friends, I also encouraged Tom to do physical activities together. He restarted playing tennis and began going on daily walks with his wife, which greatly improved the quality of their relationship. Gradually, after cardiac rehab and stepwise progression with START goals for exercise, he was able to work his way up to more than 150 minutes of moderate intensity physical activity per week.

Stress

Tom's work schedule and lack of time with family and friends made for a stressful situation. Psychosocial stress is on a par with cholesterol and blood pressure in terms of risk for heart disease. In Tom's case, he screened positive for depression. Research has shown that untreated depression can more than double one's risk for a second heart attack. In Tom's case, we worked on making lifestyle changes, using exercise as a prescription to lower stress, and I also connected him to a therapist to talk through his challenges.

Sleep

Due to his stressful work schedule, Tom was not getting enough sleep. I discussed sleep hygiene and also advised some magnesium glycinate at bedtime to help him relax further. Once we set a routine bedtime and wake-up time and began to improve his work/life balance, his sleep began to improve. The exercise was another added benefit for his sleep, in addition to the stress management techniques he learned from the therapist.

In all the components above, I worked closely with Tom, seeing him monthly, and he continued to improve in terms of his numbers, energy, and perspective on life. This is something anyone with risk factors for heart disease, or, in Tom's case, after surviving a heart attack, can do. Tom continues to do well, now having lived this healthy way for ten years after his first attack, and he says he feels more energy and joy in life than ever before.

*　　*　　*

As outlined above, anyone can benefit from applying the DRESS Code to their life, including those with chronic conditions like diabetes or heart disease. Remember, our genes do not determine our destiny. How we live our life and how we choose to engage in each of the lifestyle elements of the DRESS Code are far more important in determining both longevity and health.

As society, we need to consider policy changes that make each DRESS Code element easier for individuals to understand and optimize. For example, food policy needs to be reformed from its current state in the United States where unhealthy processed food-like substances or Frankenfoods are cheap and widely available. This makes diet a negative epigenetic input which leads to premature chronic disease and death. By shifting food policy to support local farmers to develop real, nutrient-dense food through regenerative agriculture, we can make diet a positive epigenetic input that updates our software and enables us to live our best life. The same is true for all the other lifestyle elements of the DRESS Code. Making it easier for people to move naturally and engage in physical activity will have a huge impact on both our physical and mental health. Developing communities where people gather together to connect instead of being isolated and alone will optimize the power of relationships as a key DRESS Code element in our lives. Reimagining our society in the model of the Blue Zones where the easy path is the healthy path can be particularly impactful. This has been seen with Blue Zone community projects around the country where the number of expected healthier years has increased with the changes made in these communities.

This community transformation approach needs to be paired with a health care system that prescribes food, exercise, optimal sleep, stress reduction and optimization techniques, and an encouragement of meaningful social connections as the primary approach to care. We need to go beyond simply relying on medications or surgery as our primary approach to the chronic diseases of our time that are largely determined by our lifestyle choices. While we will always need the first responder approach to acute care and medical emergencies to save lives, we need to shift upstream to prevent these chronic conditions from developing in the first place. To do this effectively, we need to allocate resources for research in the DRESS Code elements to focus medicine on lifestyle as a primary approach in health care. Furthermore, the time and expertise needed for these lifestyle prescriptions needs to be reimbursed by insurance to make it a standard part of health care so that everyone can benefit. Making these changes in health care will enable us to go from a reactive, disease-management, sick care system to a proactive, prevention and lifestyle focused, health promotion system. There is thankfully newfound awareness for this approach in Whole Person Health models of care that include the fields of integrative medicine, lifestyle medicine, culinary medicine, and functional medicine.

The goal in health care and for each of us individually should not be limited to living longer. Instead of simply striving to live longer we must learn how to live healthier for longer. Thankfully, as outlined in this book, there is no expensive technology required for us to achieve this goal. Making the changes in the DRESS Code elements are accessible, cost-effective, and practical. You don't need to know all the science behind it to benefit from the simple changes you can make every day. Like everything in life, it is a process where we will sometimes take two steps forward and one step back. As long as we continue to make lifestyle changes in each of the core DRESS Code elements, we can ultimately change the expression of our genes to keep us healthy for the long run. The key is for us to be consistent in moving forward even after any setbacks along the way. Each of us has the power to do this individually. I hope that this approach will help you to simplify longevity as something that you can understand, appreciate, and enjoy as we all strive to live our best life.

AUTHOR BIO

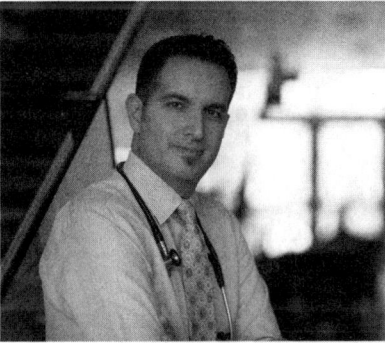

SHAD MARVASTI, MD, MPH ("Dr. Shad") is a nationally recognized leader in integrative health, culinary medicine, and lifestyle medicine. He is a Stanford-trained physician who has over two decades of experience empowering patients and communities to take charge of their health. Acting to transform and redesign medical education, he has served on the faculty at Stanford University and at The University of Arizona where he founded The Culinary Medicine Program and a Certificate of Distinction in Wellness, Integrative Medicine, and Nutrition to train future physicians with the tools they need to prevent and reverse chronic disease by addressing its root causes. He currently serves as the founding Executive Director of Whole Health and the Integrative Health and Lifestyle Medicine Institute at HonorHealth in Scottsdale, Arizona where he is developing innovative clinical models that take a whole person approach to care by realigning incentives to go from a reactive, disease management, 'sick' care system to one that is focused on keeping us healthy through a focus on prevention and the use of lifestyle interventions that proactively empower individuals and communities with the tools they need to optimize their health in all aspects of life.

Dr. Shad has been featured in national media as a trusted voice on practical, science-based wellness. His pioneering work bridges cutting-edge research with real-life application to help people live longer, healthier, and more vibrant lives.

Connect with Dr. Shad:
www.doctorshad.com
Instagram@DRSHAD9
Tik Tok@DoctorShad

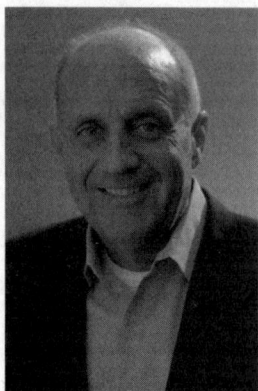

Richard H. Carmona, MD, MPH, FACS, is a renowned physician, trauma surgeon, integrative and wellness expert, and global public health leader with an extensive history of service including military, law enforcement, and public community service, he was the 17th Surgeon General of the United States. Currently, he is Chief of Health Innovations for Canyon Ranch America's preeminent health and wellness brand; he is also a Distinguished Professor of Public Health, Professor of Surgery, and Clinical Professor of Pharmacy Practice and Science at the University of Arizona; he is also a member of several Fortune 500 boards.

ENDNOTES

1   Nisha Kurani and Emma Wager, "How does the quality of the U.S. health system compare to other countries?" September 30, 2021, Peterson Center on Healthcare-KFF *Health System Tracker*, https://www.healthsystemtracker.org/chart-collection/quality-u-s-healthcare-system-compare-countries/.

2   Fani Marvasti, R. S. Stafford, "From Sick Care to Health Care—Reengineering Prevention into the U.S. System," *N Engl J Med.* 2012;367(10):889-891, doi:10.1056/NEJMp1206230https://www.ncbi.nlm.nih.gov/pmc/articles/PMC4339086/

3   WHO, *World Health Statistics: Monitoring Health for the SDGs, Sustainable Development Goals* (World Health Organization, Geneva 2020).

4   G.N. Graham, "Why Your ZIP Code Matters More Than Your Genetic Code: Promoting Healthy Outcomes from Mother to Child," Breastfeed Med, 2016 Oct;11:396-7. doi: 10.1089/bfm.2016.0113. Epub 2016 Aug 11. PMID: 27513279.

5   Dr. Kenneth R. Pelletier, *Change Your Genes, Change Your Life: Creating Optimal Health with the New Science of Epigenetics* (Origin Press, 2019).

6   Kelly M. Adams, Martin Kohlmeier, Steven H. Zeisel, "Nutrition Education in U.S. Medical Schools: Latest Update of a National Survey," *Academic Medicine*, 2010, 85(9):1537-1542. doi:10.1097/ACM.0b013e3181eab71b.

7   Kelly M. Adams, W. Scott Butsch, Martin Kohlmeier, "The State of Nutrition Education at US Medical Schools," August 6, 2015, *Journal of Biomedical Education*, https://onlinelibrary.wiley.com/doi/10.1155/2015/357627.

8   Raghupathi W, Raghupathi V. An Empirical Study of Chronic Diseases in the United States: A Visual Analytics Approach. *Int J Environ Res Public Health*. 2018;15(3):431. Published 2018 Mar 1. doi:10.3390/ijerph15030431

9   Micha R, Peñalvo JL, Cudhea F, Imamura F, Rehm CD, Mozaffarian D. Association Between Dietary Factors and Mortality From Heart Disease, Stroke, and Type 2 Diabetes in the United States. *JAMA*. 2017;317(9):912–924. doi:10.1001/jama.2017.0947

10   T. Fiolet, B. Srour, L Sellem, E. Kesse-Guyot, et al. "Consumption of Ultra-Processed Foods and Cancer Risk: Results from NutriNet-Santé Prospective Cohort BMJ 2018; 360 :k322 doi:10.1136/bmj.k322.

11   Ornish D, Lin J, Chan JM, Epel E, Kemp C, Weidner G, Marlin R, Frenda SJ, Magbanua MJM, Daubenmier J, Estay I, Hills NK, Chainani-Wu N, Carroll PR, Blackburn EH. Effect of comprehensive lifestyle changes on telomerase activity and telomere length in men with biopsy-proven low-risk prostate cancer: 5-year follow-up of a descriptive pilot study. Lancet Oncol. 2013 Oct;14(11):1112-1120. doi: 10.1016/S1470-2045(13)70366-8. Epub 2013 Sep 17. PMID: 24051140. Bottom of Form

12   Sami W, Ansari T, Butt NS, Hamid MRA. Effect of diet on type 2 diabetes mellitus: A review. *Int J Health Sci (Qassim)*. 2017;11(2):65-71.

13   The US Burden of Disease Collaborators. The State of US Health, 1990-2016: Burden of Diseases, Injuries, and Risk Factors Among US States. *JAMA*. 2018;319(14):1444–1472. doi:10.1001/jama.2018.0158

14   Health effects of dietary risks in 195 countries, 1990–2017: a systematic analysis for the Global Burden of Disease Study 2017 https://doi. org/10.1016/S0140-6736 (19)30041-8 https://www.thelancet.com/article/S0140-6736(19)30041-8/fulltext

15   Paul A.S. Breslin, An Evolutionary Perspective on Food and Human Taste, Current Biology, Volume 23, Issue 9, 2013, Pages R409-R418, ISSN 0960-9822, https://doi.org/10.1016/j.cub.2013.04.010; Diószegi Judit, Llanaj Erand, Ádány Róza, "Genetic Background of Taste Perception, Taste Preferences, and Its Nutritional Implications: A Systematic Review," Frontiers in Genetics Vol. 10, 2019. https://www.frontiersin.org/article/10.3389/fgene.2019.01272   10.3389/fgene.2019.01272

16   Baraldi LG, Martinez Steele E, Canella DS, Monteiro CA. Consumption of ultra-processed foods and associated sociodemographic factors in the USA between 2007 and 2012: evidence from a nationally representative cross-sectional study. *BMJ Open*. 2018;8(3):e020574. Published 2018 Mar 9. doi:10.1136/bmjopen-2017-020574

17   Simon Capewell, Ffion Lloyd-Williams, The role of the food industry in health: lessons from tobacco?, *British Medical Bulletin*, Volume 125, Issue 1, March 2018, Pages 131–143, https://doi.org/10.1093/bmb/ldy002

18 Wilson MM, Reedy J, Krebs-Smith SM. American Diet Quality: Where It Is, Where It Is Heading, and What It Could Be. *J Acad Nutr Diet.* 2016;116(2):302-310.e1. doi:10.1016/j.jand.2015.09.020; Mozaffarian, D., Clarke, R. Quantitative effects on cardiovascular risk factors and coronary heart disease risk of replacing partially hydrogenated vegetable oils with other fats and oils. *Eur J Clin Nutr* **63**, S22–S33 (2009). https://doi.org/10.1038/sj.ejcn.1602976; Kaur N, Chugh V, Gupta AK. Essential fatty acids as functional components of foods- a review. *J Food Sci Technol.* 2014;51(10):2289-2303. doi:10.1007/s13197-012-0677-0; Fuhrman J. The Hidden Dangers of Fast and Processed Food. *Am J Lifestyle Med.* 2018;12(5):375-381. Published 2018 Apr 3. doi:10.1177/1559827618766483

19 https://www.mic.com/articles/88015/what-happens-to-your-brain-on-sugar-explained-by-science

20 Mills S, Brown H, Wrieden W, White M, Adams J. Frequency of eating home cooked meals and potential benefits for diet and health: cross-sectional analysis of a population-based cohort study. *Int J Behav Nutr Phys Act.* 2017;14(1):109. Published 2017 Aug 17. doi:10.1186/s12966-017-0567-y

21 Julianne Holt-Lunstad, Timothy B. Smith, J. Bradley Layton, "Social Relationships and Mortality Risk: A Meta-analytic Review," July 27, 2010, *Journal of Plos Medicine,* https://doi.org/10.1371/journal.pmed.1000316.

22 Liz Mineo, "Good Genes Are Nice, But Joy Is Better," April 11, 2017, *Harvard Gazette,* https://news.harvard.edu/gazette/story/2017/04/over-nearly-80-years-harvard-study-has-been-showing-how-to-live-a-healthy-and-happy-life/.

23 Richard Weissbourd, Milena Batanova, Virginia Lovison, and Eric Torres, "Loneliness in America: How the Pandemic Has Deepened an Epidemic of Loneliness and What We Can Do About It," February 2021, Harvard Graduate School of Education, https://mcc.gse.harvard.edu/reports/loneliness-in-america.

24 Kristina Orth-Gomér, MD, PhD, Sara P. Wamala, PhD, Myriam Horsten, PhD, et al, "Marital Stress Worsens Prognosis in Women with Coronary Heart Disease," December 20, 2000, *JAMA,* https://jama-network.com/journals/jama/fullarticle/193378.

25 Michael Isiozor Nzechukwu, Setor K. Kunutsor, Tanjaniina Laukkanen, Jussi Kauhanen, and Jari A. Laukkanen, (2018). "Marriage Dissatisfaction and the Risk of Sudden Cardiac Death Among Men," January 1, 2019, *American Journal of Cardiology,* 123, 10.1016/j.amjcard.2018.09.033.

26   Laura E. Wallace, Rebecca Anthony, Christian M. End, and Baldwin M. Way, "Does Religion Stave Off the Grave? Religious Affiliation in One's Obituary and Longevity," June 13, 2018, *Social Psychological and Personality Science*, https://journals.sagepub.com/doi/10.1177/1948550618779820.

27   Jamie Ducharme, "You Asked: Do Religious People Live Longer?", February 15, 2018, *Time*, https://time.com/5159848/do-religious-people-live-longer/.

28   Ducharme, "You Asked: Do Religious People Live Longer?".

29   T. Netz, "Is the Comparison between Exercise and Pharmacologic Treatment of Depression in the Clinical Practice Guideline of the American College of Physicians Evidence-Based?, *Front Pharmaco*, 2017;8:257. Published 2017 May 15. doi:10.3389/fphar.2017.00257.

30   Siddhartha S. Angadi, Farouk Mookadam, Chong D. Lee, Wesley J. Tucker, Mark J. Haykowsky, Glenn A. Gaesser, "High-Intensity Interval Training vs. Moderate-Intensity Continuous Exercise Training in Heart Failure with Preserved Ejection Fraction: A Pilot Study," September 15, 2015, *Journal of Applied Physiology*, https://pubmed.ncbi.nlm.nih.gov/25190739/.

31   "What Is Stress?" The American Institute of Stress, https://www.stress.org/what-is-stress.

32   American Psychological Association, *Stress in America: Stress and Decision-Making During the Pandemic*, https://www.apa.org/news/press/releases/stress/2021/decision-making-october-2021.pdf.

33   https://www.cdc.gov/mmwr/preview/mmwrhtml/mm6008a2.htm#:~:text=An%20estimated%2050%2D%2D70,and%20their%20impact%20on%20health. See also https://www.cdc.gov/sleep/index.html.

34   Elizabeth Fernandez, "Lifestyle Measures May Lengthen Telomeres, A Measure of Cell Aging," September 16, 2013, University of California San Francisco, https://www.ucsf.edu/news/2013/09/108886/lifestyle-changes-may-lengthen-telomeres-measure-cell-aging.

35   T. Stockwell, J. Zhao, S. Panwar, A. Roemer, T. Naimi, T. Chikritzhs, "Do 'Moderate' Drinkers Have Reduced Mortality Risk? A Systematic Review and Meta-Analysis of Alcohol Consumption and All-Cause Mortality." J Stud Alcohol Drugs, 2016 Mar;77(2):185-98. doi: 10.15288/jsad.2016.77.185. PMID: 26997174; PMCID: PMC4803651.